The Anatomy of Injury and its Surgical Implications

The Anatomy of Injury and its Surgical Implications

P. S. London
MBE, CStJ, FRCS, MFOM, FACEM (Hon)
Honorary Consulting Surgeon to The Birmingham Accident Hospital

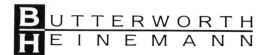

Butterworth–Heinemann Ltd
Halley Court, Jordan Hill, Oxford OX2 8EJ

 PART OF REED INTERNATIONAL P.L.C.

Oxford   London   Guildford   Boston
Munich   New Delhi   Singapore
Sydney   Tokyo   Toronto   Wellington

First published 1991   *Po4905*

© Butterworth–Heinemann Ltd, 1991

British Library Cataloguing in Publication Data
London, P. S. (Peter Stanford)
  The anatomy of injury and its surgical implications.
  1. Man. Injuries caused by accidents. Surgery
  I. Title
  617.1

  ISBN 0-75061251 7

Library of Congress Cataloging in Publication Data
Applied for

Photoset by KEYTEC, Bridport, Dorset
Printed in Great Britain by BPCC Wheatons Ltd, Exeter

Foreword

A detailed knowledge of anatomy is not a particularly good thing in itself. Committing anatomical facts to memory has little, if any, educational value, no matter what some of the old pedagogues might have thought. However, the *applications* of anatomy in clinical practice are enormously useful, not only in the obvious case of the surgeon, but also to the radiologist, neurologist and internist. Indeed, without anatomy so much of medicine remains unexplained and inexplicable.

Mr London has an international reputation as an accident surgeon of wide experience with a special flair as a teacher. In this volume he demonstrates how anatomy relates to practice in the field of accident surgery. This relationship applies to both diagnosis and treatment, and is of importance with regard to both general principles and specific injuries.

I have enjoyed reading this important contribution in manuscript. I have no doubt that its close study will benefit that 'vertebral column' of the Accident and Emergency Service – the Casualty Officer – but I equally have no doubt that his seniors will enjoy this distillation of surgical and anatomical wisdom.

Harold Ellis
Department of Anatomy,
The University of Cambridge

Introduction

Anatomy is defined as, among other things, the study of structure, particularly of the human body, and for many students that structure has been studied on preserved specimens that have been dissected for, and perhaps by, them. Anatomical textbooks have long recognized that there is more to anatomy than mere structure, by including passages on surgical and applied anatomy and, more recently, the concept of functional anatomy has been introduced. Judging by the proceedings of the Association of Clinical Anatomists, not to mention some BSc projects, the study of function has abandoned gross anatomy in favour of the use of electron microscopes and expansion into such fields as biochemistry and endocrinology.

In spite of, or perhaps because of, this extension and diversification, the newly qualified doctor is woefully ignorant of the anatomical detail that previous generations had to learn, and relies on what comes his or her way in the course of the clinical work in hand, until examination by one or other Royal College enforces detailed study of the subject. Nevertheless, even candidates for Fellowship of a Royal College of Surgeons sometimes show remarkable ignorance of what their examiners regard as basic anatomical knowledge.

Perhaps the first and one of the best opportunities for the medical student and young doctor to recognize the difference between the mere structure of the dissected specimen and the structural implications of the actions of the human body and its component parts comes in the accident and emergency department and, later, in the surgical treatment of the more serious injuries.

Active movements of the human body – the rippling muscles beloved of artists and body-builders, for example – can usually be explained by young doctors in terms of the muscles, nerves, bones and joints responsible, although facial expression or ocular movements might not be thus explained. The casualty officer and the accident surgeon are concerned not only with the effects of active movements (and with the reasons for their alteration by disease or injury) but with the effects of the application of external force. These effects can show an astonishing range that may at first sight seem to defy explanation. One example is that a fall on to the outstretched hand can produce almost any fracture or dislocation from the wrist to the shoulder. Another is the fact that whereas it is not unknown for a blow by a brick to break the fifth metacarpal bone, an exponent of karate can break a brick by hitting it with the side of his hand. The explanation lies in the prestressing effect of muscular contraction on the effective strength of bone.

It is well known that the path of a knife or bullet might be expected to have damaged this, that or the other structure, which has in fact escaped. The explanation lies in the way in which a projectile may be deflected by a bone or along a plane of cleavage provided by loose connective tissue. In addition, the fluidity of the soft tissues, aided by the lubricant effect of the loose connective tissues, enables even such seemingly delicate structures as nerves and blood vessels to be displaced from the path of a penetrating object and so to escape injury. Paré showed his understanding of the differential mobility of tissues when he succeeded in removing a musket ball from the shoulder of the Grand Master of Artillery. He succeeded after a number of others had failed because he asked the wounded man to adopt the posture in which he was at the moment of injury. This re-created the channel that had been made by the ball but that subsequently had been broken up when a change of posture caused the several layers of skin, fascia and muscle to alter their relationships.

Characteristic patterns of fracture and dislocation have their origins in the physical properties of the anatomical structures involved, although, as has just been mentioned, these can be altered by prestressing. Once this is understood, what may at first seem to be an insoluble puzzle may become susceptible to accurate analysis and may be treated successfully.

Once a bone or joint has been broken, the deformity caused by the injuring force may be replaced by that resulting from the action of both muscles and gravity on a part that has lost its stable framework. The struggles of the novice in his efforts to correct deformity may give way to the practised skill of the expert who first restores the part to the posture in which it was at the moment of injury. This process can be likened to the disengagement of two pieces of bent metal such as the puzzles that used to be put into Christmas crackers – it is easy when they are put in the appropriate relationship with each other.

These and other expressions of anatomical structure and function may be learned by those with first-hand experience of the handling of injured tissues, but a thorough understanding of these matters requires a duration and intensity of exposure that may not be provided during the years of surgical training, especially when this is confined to a particular part or system of the human body.

The advent of computed tomography has done much to add clarifying detail to the effects of injury upon both the hard and the soft tissues of the body and it may thereby raise the standard of anatomical knowledge of young doctors, at least in some respects.

Once trained, the surgeon may cease to deal with recent injuries or may deal with them only occasionally, perhaps as a matter of necessity and with little or no interest in the lessons that can still be learned – and passed on to juniors.

This subject can be thought of as the anatomy of injury or, perhaps more informatively, as the anatomy of disruption of the human body and this book is an attempt to provide practical guidance for students and young doctors engaged in the care of the injured, and food for thought for their teachers. I have, therefore, approached the subject from the point of view of the practical clinician rather than as an academic anatomist. The information has much to do with diagnosis and understanding but there are some important therapeutic applications, which are also described.

It will be noted that there are few references to published work; that is because, although much of the subject matter has appeared elsewhere at one time or another, I have written almost entirely from my own experience, although I have referred to published studies of particular importance. I have made no attempt to comb the literature for interesting rarities but I think that it is fair to say that any details gleaned from such sources would be unlikely to call in question the more general conclusions that I have recorded.

Contents

1

The head and face

Fractures of the cranium

All fractures result from a blow.

Depressed fractures

A localized blow causes a depressed fracture and often results in trapping of hair or foreign matter in the fracture line. Depressed bone may pierce the dura mater and when it lies over a venous sinus the possibility of penetration and the risk of profuse bleeding during elevation must be borne in mind when planning treatment.

Linear fractures

These result from impact over a larger area. This deforms the skull, which flattens where it is struck and becomes more sharply curved elsewhere (Evans, 1957). If this exceeds the elastic limit of the bone, the resulting linear fracture follows a more or less straight line unless it is deviated by thicker and stronger bone or into weaker parts such as sutures and thin places.

A rare type of fracture of the vault of the skull can result from a brief but powerful blow: this can split the skull and take part of it away from the dura mater as an osteoplastic flap.

Complications of fractures
Fractures of the vault of the skull

The danger of such fractures lies in the fact that they can tear veins or arteries where they lie in the path of the fissure. More or less vertical fractures of the cranium that are shown radiographically to extend to the base of the skull must be presumed to have extended into the true base of the skull, even though they are not recognized in views that show the base and even though there may at first be no supporting clinical evidence that they have done so.

Fractures of the base of the skull

These are dangerous either because they communicate with the nasal cavity, the paranasal or the mastoid sinuses and so carry the risk of meningitis or, much less often, because they tear important blood vessels. These may be in the posterior fossa, where haematomata are notoriously difficult to diagnose in good time without computed tomography, or in the region of the cavernous sinuses, thus creating a caroticocavernous fistula. The consequent back pressure leads to venous engorgement in the orbit with proptosis, pulsating exophthalmos and even blindness of the affected eye. The most severe injuries of this kind run right across the middle fossae and lead to profuse and continuing bleeding from the nose or pharynx. If there is also brain coming from the nose or the ear, there is little or no prospect that the victim will survive.

A blow on the side of the head can cause a longitudinal fracture of the petrous part of the temporal bone (Figure 1.1a). It passes through the middle ear and causes blood, but not usually cerebrospinal liquid, to escape from the ear hole. The cochlea and labyrinth may also be damaged.

A blow on the back of the head can cause a transverse fracture through the petrous bone. It passes through the labyrinth and the internal auditory meatus (Figure 1.1b), and a cerebrospinal fistula is more likely than bleeding from the ear.

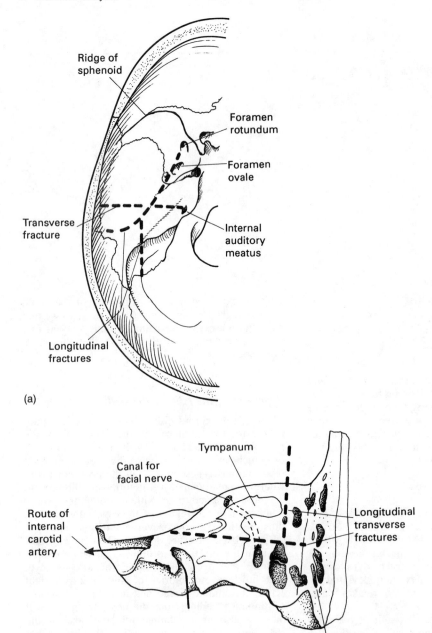

Figure 1.1. (a) The inside of the base of the skull, showing the sites of fractures of the petrous part of the temporal bone; (b) Section of the right temporal bone, showing portions of longitudinal and transverse fractures

Intracranial haematomata

The nature and effects of intracranial haematomata, particularly of extradural clots, are too well known to require description but a widespread misconception needs to be corrected. This is that death is the result of raised intracranial pressure, whereas in fact it is the result of local compression caused on the one hand by the haematoma itself and on the other by the effects of displacement and distortion of the brain (Figure 1.2), which lead to ischaemia, infarction and swelling of the brain.

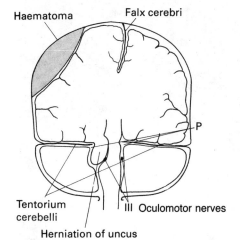

Figure 1.2. Deformation and displacement of structure within the skull caused by extradural haematoma. P: Places where pressure carries a particular risk of causing infarction

Cerebrospinal fistulae

The escape of blood or cerebrospinal liquid from the ear or the nose needs no comment, except to mention that bleeding from the ear is sometimes the result of fracture into the external auditory meatus that is caused by a blow on the point of the chin that drives the condyle of the mandible hard against the bony wall of the meatus.

Another point of interest is the presence of air within the skull. This may occur as small patches on the surface of the hemispheres but it can also take the form of large bubbles in the frontal region. These have been explained by a valvular opening through which air can be sucked from above or blown from below, but a more likely explanation is that it merely replaced pulped frontal parts of the brain that have liquefied and escaped through the fistula.

Neurological complications

Brain

A blow on the head causes movement of the brain within the skull that results in injury by impact, decompression and shearing (Pudenz and Sheldon, 1946; Strich, 1961). These events can be summarized as follows.

Because the head is supported on the hinge and pivot joints provided by the atlas and the axis, if it is struck when it is free to move it can turn, tilt and twist in response to the blow.

Because the skull and brain are for the most part separated by the narrow subarachnoid space, when the skull is set suddenly in motion by a blow it moves towards some parts of the brain and away

from others. The acceleration induced is sufficient to cause damage to the brain by both the impact (coup) and the separation (contrecoup), which latter results in what can fairly be regarded as explosive decompression. At the same time, the brain can be injured by its movement towards or away from the bony projections and the dural partitions within the skull.

A forcible blow on the head distorts the skull, which causes a sudden rise in intracranial pressure that tends to drive the brain towards the foramen magnum, and high-speed cinematography has shown a rapid sinuous deformation of the brain stem.

When the brain is set in motion by a blow on the head, the speed of motion of its parts increases with their distance from the axis of rotation and this causes shear stresses within the substance of the brain.

Cranial nerves

Olfactory nerves

The delicate filaments of these nerves are especially vulnerable to the forces that have been described.

Optic nerves

Fractures into the optic foramen can damage this nerve and cause blindness but fortunately this is rare. Even if the cause is promptly identified by computed tomography there is little prospect of saving sight by decompressing the nerve.

Oculomotor nerves

These are usually damaged by compression in the tentorial hiatus (Figure 1.2), which causes fixed dilatation of one or both pupils and paralyses all but the superior oblique and lateral rectus muscles of the eyeball. As a result, the eyeball is directed downwards and outwards.

Abducent nerves

In spite of their long course within the skull these nerves are not often injured. Paralysis of the lateral rectus muscle abolishes abduction of the eyeball.

Facial nerves

Paralysis may be immediate, because a fracture into the facial canal in the middle ear tears the nerve, or delayed, because it is compressed by local swelling.

Auditory nerves

Transverse fractures of the petrous part of the temporal bone can tear the nerve and cause deafness (Figure 1.1b). Damage to the labyrinth is rare.

Other effects of fractures

Extracranial bleeding

A simple bruise of the scalp sometimes marks the site of an extradural haematoma.

Bruising over the mastoid process is caused by blood that has tracked down from a fracture of the vault above the attachment of the temporalis muscle and emerged from beneath the galea aponeurotica.

Fractures of the occiput can cause headache and stiffness of the neck because blood tracks down among the muscles. This may suggest meningitis, or extradural or subarachnoid haemorrhage, but Kernig's sign is not present and any doubt about the conditions in the posterior fossa of the skull can be resolved by computed tomography.

Cephalhaematoma is a well-known complication of birth but massive subgaleal haematoma sometimes follows fracture of the vault later in life. The intracranial pressure is not affected by this swelling.

Surgical emphysema

Air sometimes escapes into the cheek and even into the prevertebral tissues from fracture into the maxillary sinus (Figure 1.3) and into the eyelid from fracture into the frontal sinus.

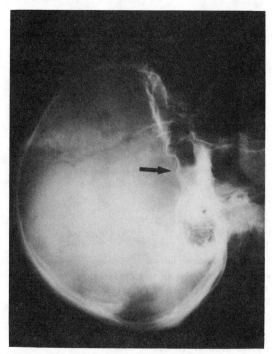

Figure 1.4. Liquid level in the sphenoidal sinus

A rare but useful sign of fracture of the base of the skull is a liquid level in the sphenoidal sinus (Figure 1.4). This is worth looking for in any lateral view of the skull after head injury and it is most easily recognized if the film is examined with the brow uppermost.

Fractures of the face and orbits

Middle third of the face

The classic experiments of Le Fort (1901) demonstrated the main patterns of fractures of this part and how they are related to its weak regions (Figure 1.5).

Nose

A blow from the side pushes the nose sideways and may jam one nasal bone beneath the other (Figure 1.6a). When this happens the deformity cannot be corrected until the depressed bone has been lifted out of the way. Correction is achieved by a twisting with Walsham's forceps on each of the two bones.

A blow from the front flattens the nose and crumples the septum; correction requires a lifting action (when the patient is supine), the effects of which are prolonged by a stitch passed through the nose from side to side, and an external splint

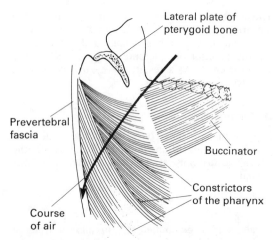

Figure 1.3. Air escaping from a crack in the back of the maxillary sinus has a continuous plane of cleavage round the constrictions of the pharynx to the prevertebral fascia

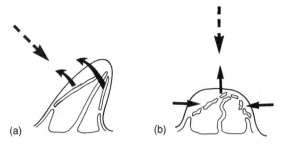

Figure 1.6. (a) Pushover fracture of the nose; (b) the flattened nose. Corrective forces are shown by solid arrows and injuring forces by dotted arrows

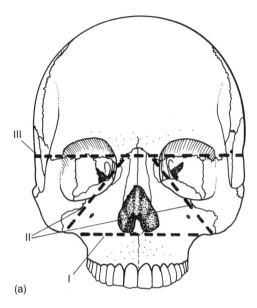

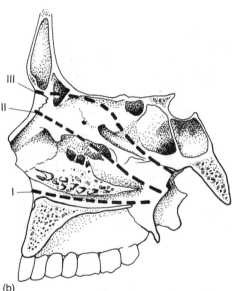

Figure 1.5. The middle third of the face and its fractures (a) Le Fort's 3 patterns of fractures; (b) sagittal section through the nasal cavity and pharynx to show the positions of Le Fort's fractures. It will be noted that when the central block of bone is displaced backwards it can block the nasopharynx

(Figure 1.6b). Blood may collect on one or both sides between the septal cartilage and its perichondrium; unless it is promptly drained this may kill the cartilage, which later crumples, causing deformity of the nose.

Zygomatic bone

A blow on the cheek can drive the strong cortical block of the body of the bone into the thin-walled maxillary sinus, with accompanying fractures in or near the adjoining frontal and temporal bones (Figure 1.5a). The depression is quickly masked by swelling of the soft tissues unless the bony contours are carefully compared by palpation as well as by inspection. Looking down from above and using the eyebrows for reference is particularly helpful if the tips of the index fingers are pressed firmly against the summits of the bodies of the zygomatic bones. Blood tracks down into the cheek to accentuate the bulge above and behind the angle of the mouth on that side and it tracks upwards and forwards beneath the conjunctiva. Bleeding into the maxillary sinus may overflow into the nasal cavity and thence from the nostril on the injured side. The infraorbital nerve, which supplies branches to the upper lip and the incisor teeth, may be damaged where it lies in the infra-orbital canal.

Computed tomography shows the details clearly but, in whatever combination, the physical signs, together with a graze or bruise over the cheekbone, are often more reliable than radiography for diagnosing the fracture.

The 'blow-out' fracture is a special sort of fracture affecting the floor of the orbit (to which the zygomatic bone contributes). A blow in the eye, particularly by a squash ball, which seals the orbit, produces a high enough pressure within it to blow out part of the floor into the maxillary sinus; the eyeball therefore looks sunken and its movements are affected by damage to, or displacement of, the inferior oblique and inferior rectus muscles.

Fracture of the zygomatic arch results from a blow on it. Sometimes the indentation is sufficient to foul the temporalis muscle and the coronoid process of the mandible and so interfere with opening the mouth and sideways movements of the lower jaw.

Therapeutic implications

Many fractures of the zygomatic bone will stay in place when they have been elevated; this should be tested at the time of elevation so that surgical fixation or packing of the maxillary sinus can be undertaken if simple elevation fails. Elevation is greatly facilitated by the fact that the temporal fascia is attached to the zygomatic arch. Once passed through a cut in the fascia (not the temporalis muscle), the elevating tool is easily directed beneath the body of the bone (Figure 1.7).

It will be noted that the optic foramen is well away from these fractures (Figure 1.5); nevertheless, blindness has been known to occur in some cases. It is therefore important to test vision before undertaking any treatment that might otherwise be blamed.

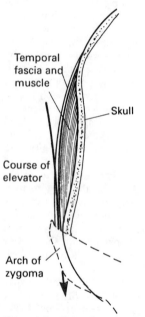

Temporal fascia and muscle

Skull

Course of elevator

Arch of zygoma

Figure 1.7. Coronal section showing the guiding role of the temporal fascia

Fractures of the mandible

The patterns of the fractures are determined in the first place by the site and direction of the blow. Once the bone has been broken, displacement of the fragments depends on the shape of the fracture and the action of muscles (Figure 1.8). Surgical fixation is necessary in most cases. Because it runs within the bone, the inferior dental nerve is damaged by many fractures; it supplies the lower teeth and part of the skin of the chin.

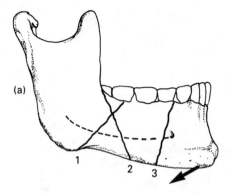

(a)

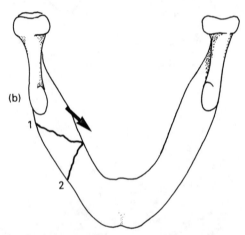

(b)

Figure 1.8. Fractures of the mandible, to show the displacing effects of the muscles attached to it. Fracture 1; The muscles attached to the proximal fragment act generally in the direction of the arrow and will tend to open it, whereas fracture 2 will tend to be closed. When fracture 3 affects both sides, the anterior fragment will be pulled downwards and backwards. The dotted line marks the course of the inferior dental nerve within the bone

Teeth may be cracked, broken off or displaced from their sockets; an empty socket should prompt a search to show whether or not a tooth has been inhaled.

Injuries of the soft tissues

Scalp

It is well known that a blow on the scalp with a blunt object can split it so cleanly as to suggest that it has been cut.

A blow at an acute angle to the surface can create a flap by splitting the scalp and separating it from the galea aponeurotica through the loose connective between them. Avulsion of the scalp is now rare; it occurs through the same plane of cleavage and may extend as far as the eyebrows, the ears and the nape of the neck.

Face

Eyelids

Wounds of the lids occur fairly often but are rarely dangerous. This is partly because, when the lids are closed tightly in reaction to a threat, there is nearly half an inch (≈13 mm) of tissue in front of the eyeball. Danger may arise when a wound follows a fall, or may for other reasons be of a penetrating nature, and affects the medial part of the upper lid: the danger lies in the possibility that the wound has pierced the thin roof of the orbit and even the brain (Figure 1.9). The converse of this injury is a fracture of the floor of the anterior fossa of the skull that opens into the nasal cavity. It has been known for a nasogastric tube to pass through it and enter the cranial cavity.

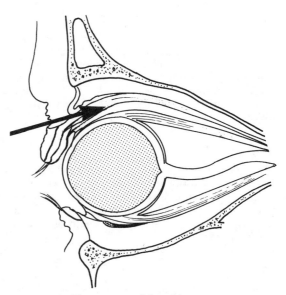

Figure 1.10. The contents of the orbit

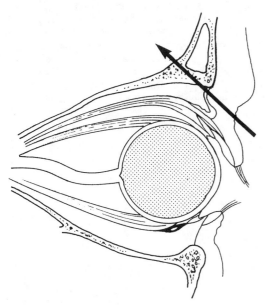

Figure 1.9. Diagram to show the route from the upper lid to the anterior fossa of the skull

Foreign bodies in the orbit

The fact that a hammer can dislodge from the mushroomed head of a chisel a flake of metal that can penetrate the eyeball has often been recorded but it is still not sufficiently well known by junior casualty officers. It is perhaps even less well known that fragments from a shattered windscreen, for example, can enter the orbit without necessarily damaging the eye. Figure 1.10 shows the relevant structure of the orbit and its contents. The orbital fascia (periosteum) is fairly loosely attached to the bone and can be regarded as the outermost layer of a sheath of fascia, muscles and fat that surrounds the eyeball and the optic nerve. When the lids are closed, fragments following the course of the arrow can enter the orbit between the superior tarsal plate and the bony roof of the orbit. Their presence within the orbit can displace the eye forwards and may stretch or distort the optic nerve but, being blunt and travelling fairly slowly, they remain outside the aforementioned sheath and do no direct damage to the structures inside it. Initial impairment of vision can be followed by complete recovery if the eyeball is allowed promptly to regain its natural position in the orbit.

Skin of the face

A rare but horrifying injury occurs when the face is subjected to a violent shearing force that tears away more or less of the skin and fat from the fascia and muscles beneath. In severe cases, when the resulting flap is straightened out the examiner may find himself looking out between the victim's lips. Fortunately, there is usually a large enough attachment for the flap to remain alive.

Pinna

The pinna owes its shape to its core of fibrocartilage; this is nourished by its perichondrium and is encased by skin.

Haematoma

A blow on the ear can cause bleeding between the cartilage and the perichondrium and results in a thick ear. Unless the blood is promptly evacuated and the perichondrium is allowed (by continuous suction – compression is not enough) to grow back on to the cartilage, the latter will die and shrivel, which results in a cauliflower ear.

Avulsion

If the pinna is pulled or is subjected to a shearing force it can be torn away from the scalp. The skin splits and the cartilage is pulled out. If the flap so formed retains an adequate blood supply it is sufficient to tuck the cartilage back into place and sew up the skin.

Lips

A blow on the lip can split it more or less cleanly against the teeth but if the blow is at an acute angle to the surface it can shear the lip, sometimes extensively, from its attachment to the gum.

Children's lips are quite often bitten by dogs. A slashing action by a canine tooth may do no more than split the lip cleanly but sometimes part of one or both lips is bitten off as they are pursed – the so-called kiss bite, which is characteristically ragged.

Fauces

A child that falls with a stick in its mouth may be seen to have a tear in or near the tonsillar fossa. This should not be dismissed lightly because the internal carotid artery is close by and has been known to suffer traumatic thrombosis (Figure 1.11).

The importance of knowing the details of the circumstances in which the injuries illustrated by Figure 1.10 as well as by Figure 1.11 occurred is obvious. All falls and blows, whether deliberate or accidental, must be regarded as forcible injuries, with due regard to the structures at risk.

References

Evans, F. G. (1957) *Stress and Strain in Bones, their Relation to Fractures and Osteogenesis,* Thomas, Springfield

Le Fort, R. (1901) Etude experimentale sur les fractures de la machoire supérieure. *Revue Chirurgicale,* **23**, 8

Pudenz, R. H. and Sheldon, C. H. (1946) The lucite calvarium – a method for direct observation of the brain, cranial trauma and brain movement. *Journal of Neurosurgery,* **3**, 487

Strich, S. J. (1961) Shearing of nerve fibres as a cause of brain damage due to head injury. Lancet, **ii**, 443

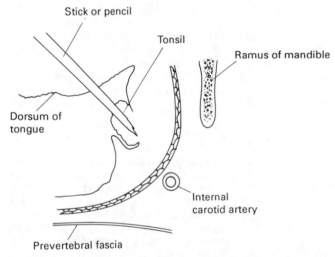

Figure 1.11. Cross section of the oropharynx and adjoining structures

2

The neck

The shape of the head and much of the face is fixed by the skull but in the neck the soft tissues make up most of its bulk and this part of the spine is more flexible than any other. A clear understanding of how these structures react to injurious stresses is of great assistance both in making a diagnosis and in planning treatment.

Bones and joints

Apart from penetrating injuries, the cervical spine is injured by movements of flexion, extension and rotation and also by end-to-end compression. Flexion and extension result from energy transmitted from either the body or the head and these methods of transmission are referred to here as, respectively, inertial movements and direct force.

Injuries by inertial movements

These occur when the body is either accelerated or decelerated in relation to the head when the head is free to move. They are more often movements of extension than of flexion. When a stationary vehicle is run into from behind, the body is accelerated from rest and the head is, as it were, left behind, with the result that there is sudden extension of the head and neck. This is often referred to as a whiplash injury but an extension sprain is a more accurate and informative term. It may be painful but it is not usually serious, although its profitable consequences are becoming more widely known and exploited in courts of law.

The opposite movement of flexion stops when the chin reaches the chest, and it usually causes no trouble. It has been found, however, that the violence resulting from rapid vertical descent in a crashing aircraft can cause fracture of the sternum and damage to the heart in this way, but the victims are usually killed by other injuries.

Injuries by direct force: extension

In later life the neck is particularly vulnerable by sudden extension, with the result that a blow in the face or brow can cause serious and even fatal damage. It can break the odontoid process of the axis, avulse the anterior longitudinal ligament and break the posterior part of the arch of the atlas (Figure 2.1). The cause of the fracture of the odontoid process is presumably avulsion by the strong alar ligaments that attach the tip of the process to the base of the skull. Although in theory the process might be broken by impact by the front of the arch of the atlas, the relative strengths of the two bones makes this unlikely; furthermore, when the atlas is broken by extension the fracture is at the back, not the front of the ring.

The spinal cord usually escapes damage and the support of a firm collar is often sufficient treatment. Another result of forcible extension of the neck of an elderly person occurs when there are degenerative changes. As the intervertebral discs lose their resilience the lowest ones flatten and bulge into the vertebral canal by one-quarter inch (≈ 6 mm) or more (Figure 2.1). Sudden extension causes the soft tissues between the neural arches to bulge forwards and these posterior bulges are opposite the ones in front. It should be remembered that this part of the spine contains the cervical enlargement of the spinal cord, which further reduces the space available for any encroachment to occur without causing harm.

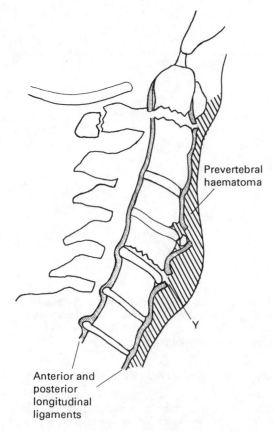

Figure 2.1. Sagittal section to show some effects of forcible extension of the neck. Y, an injury that occurs in young adults, often without fracture

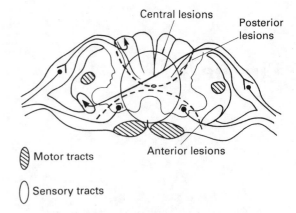

Figure 2.2. Cross-section of the spinal cord. Posterior lesions affect mainly fine touch and proprioception; central lesions cause partial paralysis and affect perception of temperature and touch because their tracts cross from one side of the cord to the other; anterior lesions affect mainly motor pathways and cells in the motor horns of the grey matter

The effect of these bulges may be to damage the front, the centre or, rarely, the back of the spinal cord. Sometimes there is complete paralysis but the most usual result is an upper motor neurone lesion affecting the lower limbs, which recover more or less, and a lower motor neurone lesion that affects the hands (Figure 2.2) and is permanent.

Young spines can also be damaged by extension but it has to be much more forcible than in the elderly. Congenital anomalies that reduce the flexibility of the spine, and ankylosing spondylitis, increase its vulnerability to flexion as well as extension. Rheumatoid arthritis and mongolism weaken the ligaments and so put the spine at risk.

Occipitoatlantic dislocation

This rare but not necessarily fatal result of forcible extension gives substance to the threat, 'I'll knock your block off'. Post-mortem dissection has shown that all or most of the ligaments have been torn

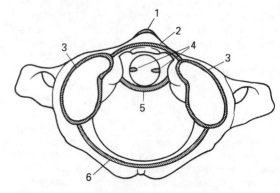

Figure 2.3. The ligaments attached to the atlas as seen from above: 1, anterior longitudinal ligament; 2, anterior atlantooccipital membrane; 3, capsules of synovial joints; 4, alar ligaments; 5, transverse ligament of the atlas; 6, posterior atlantooccipital membrane

(Figure 2.3) (Bucholz and Burkhead, 1979). Associated injuries of the face have suggested that rotation as well as extension can play a part in causing this injury (Evarts, 1970; Page *et al.*, 1973).

Hangman's fracture

Hyperextension combined with traction breaks the pedicles of the axis and disrupts the disc between the second and third cervical vertebrae. The forward displacement that is shown radiographically suggests that this injury is caused by flexion but the displacement results from the effects of gravity on the damaged joint. Although this injury results from judicial execution by hanging, when inflicted accidentally, often in a road accident, there may be little or no neural damage.

Hyperextension tears

A third effect of forcible extension that sometimes occurs in young spines is less familiar to clinicians than to morbid anatomists because there may be no radiologically evident bony damage and the victim often dies without regaining consciousness. The anterior longitudinal ligament is torn and the tear extends backwards between the body of a vertebra and the intervertebral disc (Figure 2.1, Y). Good lateral views of the neck are an essential component of the initial examination of the victims of head injury and if they are examined carefully, chip fractures of the articular facets or of the front of the body of a vertebra or swelling of the soft tissues in front of the spine may be seen (Figure 2.1) when this injury has occurred. Computed tomography would show the damage clearly but the unaided clinician may be able to diagnose the lesion (but must first suspect it) by passing a finger down the throat. When they are present, the boggy swelling, the gap and the abnormal mobility are easy to feel.

Comment

The level at which the neck is injured depends on where the blow lands, its direction and perhaps its duration. It depends also on the state of the muscles, which can exert a strong protective effect on bone when they are contracted. These details are often a matter of speculation in the individual case but even slight evidence of injury of the front of the face or brow should prompt a deliberate clinical and radiological search for the possible effects in the spine, the spinal cord and its nerve roots.

Injury by direct force: flexion

The cause is a heavy blow from behind that forces the neck into flexion; it often has components of twisting and compression as well. Such a force is exerted by a fall onto the head or the shoulders from a tree, from a crashing vehicle, by diving into shallow water or on landing badly on a trampoline or after a high jump. The neck can also be forced into flexion in a loose or a set scrum or in a head-on tackle in Rugby football. What happened is usually clear from the account given by the patient, a witness or a combination of the circumstances and any marks of impact.

Occipitoatlantic dislocation

Forwards displacement of the head (Gabrielsen and Maxwell, 1966; Page *et al.*, 1973) may not damage the spinal cord but in Gabrielsen and Maxwell's patient the greater occipital nerve was injured. Apart from a collar for comfort, the only treatment was late fusion because of clicking and anxiety. This injury is rare and, judging from accompanying injuries of the face, some examples of it may have been the result of extension with subsequent displacement by gravity.

Atlantoaxial injuries

Anterior displacement of the atlas is usually accompanied by fracture of the odontoid process of the axis; less often, the axis remains unbroken but the transverse ligament of the atlas ruptures. This is a much more dangerous injury because of the possibility that the spinal cord will be crushed (Figure 2.4).

As with fractures caused by extension, the odontoid process is most probably pulled off by the alar ligaments that connect it with the skull.

Diagnostic difficulties

Injuries of this part of the spine are notoriously easy to overlook; casualty officers, in particular, should be trained to examine radiographs of the area with great care in all cases, whether or not there is any reason to suspect that it has been injured. The features of the lateral views have been indicated and are sometimes fairly obvious, whereas those of the anteroposterior views are often much less obvious and may be blurred by the upper incisor teeth or confused by the effects of rotation.

The following arrangements should be examined carefully and if there is any suspicion of injury, suitable advice should be sought without delay.

In Figure 2.5, on each side, (1) is the distance between the side of the odontoid process and the inner border of the lateral mass of the atlas; (2) is the distance between the side of the odontoid process and the inner margin of the inferior articular facet of the axis and (3) is the congruity of the lateral atlantoaxial joints.

Figure 2.5a shows the normal appearance with the head looking forwards; Figure 2.5b is the normal appearance when the head is turned to the left; (1) is unequal on the two sides, (2) remains equal and the displacement of (3) is equal and in the same direction on the two sides. This appearance is likely to be present when the neck is too stiff and painful for the radiographer to obtain a true anteroposterior view.

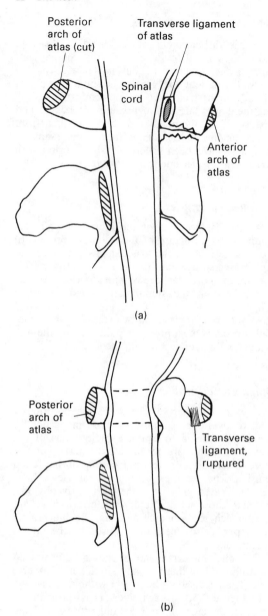

Figure 2.4. Sagittal section to show the differences between dislocation of the atlas (a) with and (b) without fracture of the odontoid process of the axis

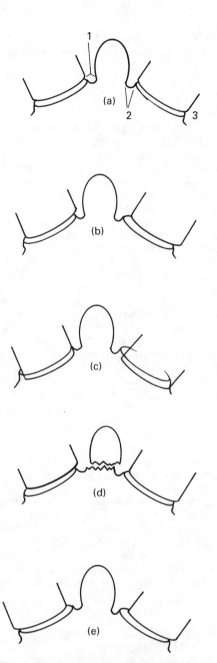

Figure 2.5. Normal and abnormal appearances of the atlantoaxial joint as shown radiographically

In Figure 2.5c, (1) is unequal on the two sides, (2) is equal, (3) shows overlapping facets, with those of the atlas displaced equally in the same direction. This is the result of atlantoaxial dislocation without fracture.

In Figure 2.5d, (1) is equal, (2) is unequal and (3) shows equal displacement in the same direction. This is the result of atlantoaxial fracture-dislocation.

In Figure 2.5e, (1) may be equal or not but is increased on both sides, (2) is equal and (3) shows displacements that may be equal or unequal but are in opposite directions. This is the result of fracture of the ring of the atlas in two places (burst fracture). The slope of occipitoatlantic joints allows a blow on the top of the head to drive the sides of the atlas apart.

Flexion injuries below the axis

In children, an anterior step between the second and the third cervical vertebrae is normal but it is sometimes mistaken for a subluxation; the backs of the vertebral bodies, the articular masses and the neural arches retain their proper relationships but the amount of cartilage in a young spine may not make this easy to recognize.

In adults, mildly torn ligaments may not be accompanied by fractures and may at first allow little displacement. Unless computed tomography is used, such injuries are easily overlooked until persistent complaints lead to further radiological examination and forwards subluxation is found to have occurred. If the injury is suspected at the beginning and the neck is radiographed in flexion and extension, muscular spasm (or, to use a more accurate term, protective muscular activity) may hold the vertebrae together.

Tell-tale signs (Figure 2.6) are:

1. Slight discontinuity in the line of the backs of the vertebral bodies; the corresponding line in front may not be affected at first.
2. Slight loss of congruity of the articular facets. Computed tomography, but not usually plain radiographs, may show small chip fractures.

The gaps between the spinous processes vary so much, even in the same person, that they are of little or no diagnostic use.

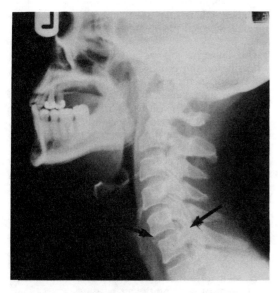

Figure 2.6. Mild subluxation without fracture. The small bony shadow in front of the subluxation was not of recent origin. The questing and discerning eye will recognize the slight displacement indicated by the arrow. Note the variation in the sizes and spacing of the spinous processes

A mild injury of this sort tears the capsules of the synovial joints; once they have given way, some subluxation can take place even though the ligamentum nuchae and the posterior longitudinal ligaments are intact.

Dislocated facets occur when there has been more severe and extensive tearing of the ligaments of the spine. The ligamenta flava and capsules are torn where the dislocation occurs; elsewhere, the ligamentum nuchae and the longitudinal ligaments are peeled from the bone or merely stretched. When both facets are dislocated the deformity is radiologically obvious but both the spinal cord and the nerve roots can escape injury, even late in life. The anterior step amounts to half or more of the anteroposterior dimension of the vertebral body. Careful examination of the radiographs will reveal that the lateral masses of each vertebra are superimposed at each level. Small fractures may occur but they can be ignored unless they render the spine unstable after the dislocation has been corrected.

A combination of flexion and rotation causes one facet to ride up over the one below and then lock in front of it, perhaps pressing on the nerve root. When only one facet has been dislocated the fact may not be recognized; this is because the condition is not seen very often in the average casualty department and neither the physical nor the radiological signs are obvious early on. Nevertheless, an astute doctor should be able to suspect the condition on clinical grounds and confirm it with plain radiographs:

1. The injury most often occurs in young adults.
2. There is a history of a fall or wrench, after which the neck becomes stiff and painful.
3. Pain and perhaps weakness and numbness may be present at once in the distribution of the nerve root that has been affected but sometimes these symptoms come on after an interval that ranges from minutes to hours and they may not be reported by the patient.
4. The head and neck may be held at an unusual angle but if the victim is lying down this may go unrecognized until the radiographer tries to obtain true anteroposterior and lateral views of the neck.

Once aroused, suspicion should direct attention to the possibility of sensory changes and abnormal radiographic appearances. Although deformity is most easily recognized in special oblique views, which show elongation of the normally circular intervertebral foramen and reversal of the natural positions of the articular facets, the discerning eye will find the necessary evidence in the plain lateral view (Figure 2.7). The anteroposterior view shows a break in the line of the spinous processes. Chip fractures may be present but demonstrable only by computed tomography.

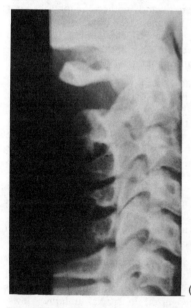

(a)

(b)

Figure 2.7. a, The characteristic appearance of dislocation of one facet as shown by a lateral view of the spine. The step is not more than about one-quarter of the anteroposterior dimension of the body of the vertebra and there are two columns of facets above the lesion but only one column (because of superimposition) below it. b, Lateral view after correction of the dislocation. A small step remains but the facets are now superimposed above the lesion as well as below it

Implications for treatment

These are important. The role of flexion, rotation and compression in causing these injuries makes obvious the need for traction, rotation and extension for correcting deformity but a warning is necessary. The fact that extension of the head helps to clear the air passages, particularly in an unconscious person, does not mean that it is in all cases safe to extend the head; in some cases the neck has been injured by extension. Furthermore, when both facets have been dislocated by a flexion force, extension of the neck while the joints are still dislocated can injure the spinal cord by accentuating existing distortion. The dilemma cannot be resolved completely but its existence should be known to doctors and other advanced first-aiders.

It may fairly be recommended that if the victim of known or suspected injury of the neck is breathing easily it is sufficient to provide firm, comfortable support for the head and neck by means of a collar or sandbags and continue to observe the breathing. If breathing is obstructed one can safely lift the lower jaw forwards, pull the tongue forwards or extend the head on the neck while at the same time pulling gently on it. As far as possible, the neck should not be extended. Whether in hospital or at the roadside, urgent intubation of the trachea should as far as possible take account of the dangers of extension but if the worst comes to the worst, imminent death from suffocation takes priority over the risk of damaging the spinal cord.

Radiographers may need supervision and assistance in their efforts to obtain good views of the neck.

The dangerous effects of twisting the neck have a bearing on the process of turning a person over and the use of the so-called recovery position. The joint first aid manual of the St John Ambulance Association, the British Red Cross Society and the St Andrew's Ambulance Association gives detailed instructions about how to safeguard the spinal cord but however suitable for trained and experienced persons these instructions may be, they are likely to overtax the anxious first-aider who is trying in an emergency to explain to others what to do and how to do it.

The simplest advice to give is as follows:

1. Think of the possibility that the neck has been injured.
2. Try to maintain the position of the head and neck relative to the trunk, especially when moving the patient or clearing the air passages.
3. No collar or other appliance available to first-aiders immobilizes the neck, it merely supports it.

It has to be admitted, however, that this advice is more easily given than taken.

The recovery position is liable to twist the neck, particularly in the course of an ambulance journey, in which the body may be swung and swayed a good deal.

Injury by direct force: compression

Like rotation, compression plays some part in causing most fractures of the neck, but there is a group of injuries in which compression is the dominant force. Within this group the compression may or may not be combined with flexion.

Simple compression

Compression without flexion occurs when the spine is in a more or less straight line. It causes a bursting injury of the vertebral body(ies). Except when it affects the atlas, it endangers the spinal cord (Figure 2.8). In the anteroposterior view a vertical split in the body of a vertebra must be distinguished from air in the larynx (Figure 2.9).

Compression with flexion

This crushes the front of the vertebral column; it often does little or no damage to the back (Figure

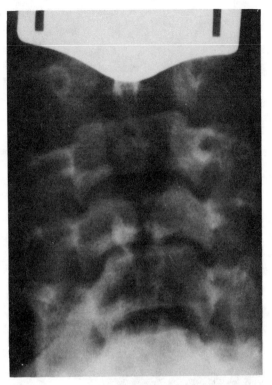

Figure 2.9. Air in the larynx overlying a vertical split in the body of a vertebra. (By courtesy of Dr Victor Pullicino)

2.10) with the result that the spinal cord and its nerves escape injury but it can be of such violence that it displaces the body of a vertebra backwards and so crushes the cord.

Other types of compression injury are less frequent and can result in isolated fractures of articular facets.

Injury by traction

Chips of bone are quite often pulled off by ligaments but they may not be shown by ordinary radiographs. Perhaps the best known, but rather rare, example of a traction fracture is the so-called clay shoveller's fracture, in which the tip of the spinous process of the seventh cervical vertebra is pulled off by muscular action. Horizontal fractures through spinous processes (Chance's fractures) sometimes accompany dislocation of facets.

Soft tissues

Closed injuries

These result from compression or more or less forcible blows.

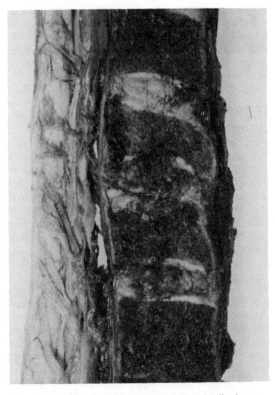

Figure 2.8. Bursting injury caused by longitudinal compression of the spine; tetraplegia resulted

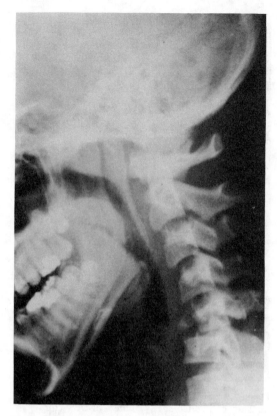

Figure 2.10. Compression with flexion that did not tear ligaments or injure the spinal cord, in spite of the step

Fracture of the hyoid bone

This bone can reasonably be considered with the soft tissues that are attached to it. Fracture is almost always the result of manual strangulation; the greater cornua of the bone are easily felt and are vulnerable in this way.

Larynx and trachea

Most of the structures in the neck are sufficiently mobile and flexible to 'ride' a blow but the greater rigidity and fixity of the larynx and trachea render them vulnerable, particularly by a blow on the front of the neck (Figure 2.11). If the larynx is forced back against the spine, being open at the back, it is liable to split vertically whereas the trachea is usually torn across, partly or completely, between the rings of cartilage. Sometimes it is detached from the larynx. These injuries are rare but there may be good reasons for suspecting them.

1. There may be a history of a forcible blow on the front of the neck, quite likely in a road accident.

2. Spotty bruising means that the skin has been driven hard against the spine. There may well be ordinary bluish bruising and also grazing but these signs do not have the same ominous significance as purplish-brown spots on skin that does not lie directly over bone. They can fairly be likened to the pattern on a coin or medal, which requires a heavy blow and unyielding support for what is struck. In the neck, and elsewhere, the unyielding support provided by the spine is several layers of tissue away from the point of impact and some of those intervening tissues are liable to be injured.

3. There may be difficulty in breathing and perhaps cyanosis.

4. There may be surgical emphysema in the neck. At first this may be evident to the fingers rather than to the eye but it can become massive and extensive.

In severe cases, if intubation of the trachea is impossible, tracheotomy is urgently required.

Wounds of the neck

Wounds of the neck are mostly caused by cutting or by penetrating objects.

Cut throat

Persons attempting suicide usually throw the head well back before cutting the throat; this brings the trachea and adjoining structures further forwards, with the result that the cut has to be very much deeper than most are if it is to cut the main blood vessels.

Penetrating wounds

The differential mobility of the soft tissues of the neck means that the path of a penetrating object is not necessarily a straight line from the point of entry to the point of exit or lodgement as shown by radiographs. Stab wounds do little or no damage to important structures in up to 50% of cases and an experienced surgeon will not explore all such wounds. The explanation of the fact that important structures often escape damage is illustrated by Figure 2.12. Once the weapon has pierced the skin this may slide along it and stain it with blood for a few inches from the tip, which is then resting between structures that have come into contact with it quite gently and have not been damaged by it. It should, however, be remembered that a penetrating object may have been stopped by contact with the spine and that radiographs should be inspected carefully for evidence that one or more vertebrae have been injured.

Exploration should be undertaken when there is evidence of injury to important structures, as indicated by the following:

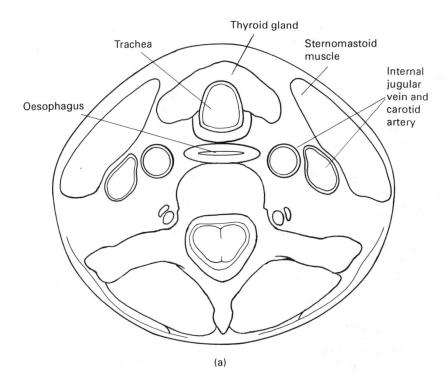

(a)

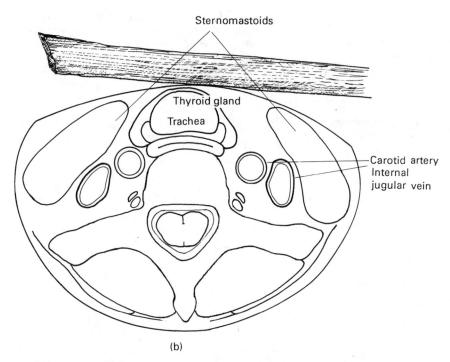

(b)

Figure 2.11. The effect of a blow on the front of the neck. The muscles and main blood vessels are protected in the angles between the body of the vertebra and the transverse processes, whereas the larynx and trachea can be crushed against the spine

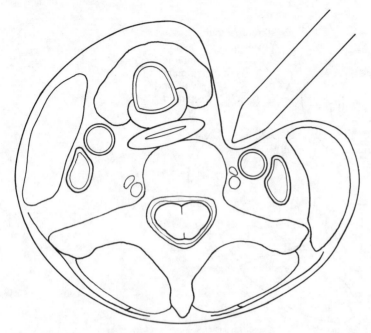

Figure 2.12. Cross-section of the neck to show how its structures can be displaced before the skin is pierced by a sharp object

1. Profuse or continuing external bleeding
2. Haemoptysis
3. Alteration of the voice
4. Difficulty in swallowing
5. Evidence of paralysis, e.g. Horner's syndrome
6. Escape of watery liquid, food or air from the wound
7. Gas bubbles near the air passages or the oesophagus
8. Haemothorax
9. Large or rapidly expanding pneumothorax; the dome of the pleura rises about an inch above the clavicle in an upright adult.

References

Bucholz, R. W. and Burkhead, W. Z. (1979) The pathological anatomy of fatal atlanto-occipital dislocations. *Journal of Bone and Joint Surgery*, **61A**, 248

Evarts, C. M. (1970) Traumatic occipito-atlantal dislocation. *Journal of Bone and Joint Surgery*, **52A**, 1653

Gabrielsen, T. O. and Maxwell, J. A. (1966) Traumatic atlanto-occipital dislocation. *American Journal of Roentgenology*, **97** 624

Page, C. P., Story, J. L., Wissinger, J. P. and Branch, C. L. (1973) Traumatic atlantooccipital dislocation: case report. *Journal of Neurosurgery*, **39**, 394

3

The shoulder girdle

Fractures and dislocations

Most of these result from a blow or a fall. Figure 3.1 shows the general directions of the most frequent injuring forces acting on the shoulder girdle. Arrows 1, 2, 3 and 4 represent direct impact and arrow 5 represents force directed along the humerus.

Scapula

Force 1 causes a fracture of the body of the scapula. Although at the moment of impact the fragments may be quite widely scattered, as shown radiographically, they are usually fairly close together and, being well clad by muscles with a good blood supply, they unite rapidly, regardless of treatment.

Force 2 causes fracture of the acromion process or the spine of the scapula just medial to it; both are rare and usually unite without trouble.

Force 3 drives the head of the humerus against the glenoid surface of the scapula and either bone can break. Great force can shatter both, otherwise the glenoid is likely to break across below its middle but this is not a frequent injury.

Shoulder joint

Force 4. When the arm is by the side, a blow directed forwards against the head of the humerus may knock it out of joint but anterior dislocation occurs more often when the arm is raised above shoulder height, as when falling on to the outstretched hand (Figure 3.1b). In this case, force is

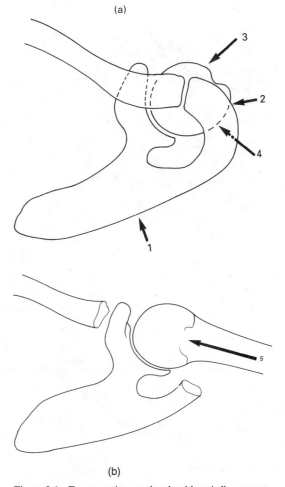

Figure 3.1. Forces acting on the shoulder girdle, as seen from above

directed along the line of the humerus, of which the head takes the line of least resistance, downwards and forwards below the coracoacromial arch (Figure 3.2a). The inclination of the glenoid surface of the scapula means that, relative to the angle of the scapula, the direction of the dislocating force is not all that much different from that of force 4.

Although Kocher's and Hippocrates' methods of replacing a dislocated shoulder have stood the test of time, they are not without complications. Anatomically, the most natural manoeuvre is to reverse force 5 in Figure 3.1b by abducting and flexing the shoulder and then pulling on the arm and pushing the head of the humerus upwards. Indeed, spontaneous replacement sometimes occurs when a patient lies prone on a couch with the dislocated shoulder projecting from it and the upper limb hanging straight down.

Anterior dislocation   may be accompanied by fracture of the greater tuberosity, the head of the humerus or the rim of the glenoid. The greater tuberosity is sheared off against the edge of the glenoid and it often retains its attachment to both the rotator cuff and the periosteum. As a result, when the head of the humerus is replaced, its tuberosity may also resume its place. If the periosteum has been torn, however, the pull of the rotator cuff can tilt the fragment on edge and so interfere with movement of the joint unless it is replaced surgically.

The impact of the head of the humerus with the edge of its bony socket can either dent the back of the head or break off the anteroinferior rim of the socket. Whether or not these fractures occur, and

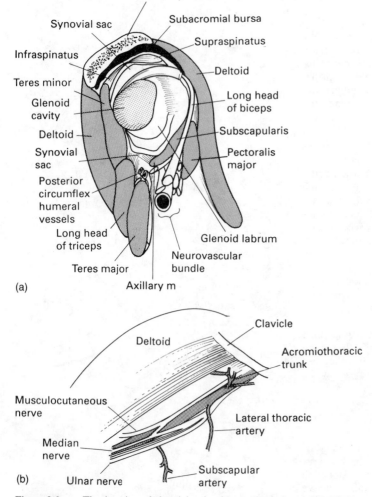

(a)

(b)

Figure 3.2. a, The interior of the right shoulder as seen from the side; b, the neurovascular bundle in front of the shoulder joint

which of them, depends on the precise direction of the injuring force and the relationship of the bones at the moment of injury.

Figure 3.2b shows the relationship of the main neurovascular bundle to the shoulder. The vulnerability of the axillary nerve by anterior dislocation is well known but it is less well known that paralysis of the deltoid muscle prevents neither the initiation nor the completion of the movement of abduction at the shoulder. Nor is it as well known as it should be that the rest of the brachial plexus in this region is at risk and that any part, or the whole of it, can be injured. Feeling and movement therefore need to be tested throughout the upper limb.

Damage to the axillary or to the brachial artery is more likely when the vessel is stiffened by atherosclerosis in later life. Occasionally the subscapular artery is torn; this can lead to marked swelling and bruising in the axilla and of the adjoining part of the chest wall but it may not obliterate the radial pulse at the wrist.

Posterior dislocation is much rarer than anterior and it is characteristically the result of inward rotation and posterior displacement of the humerus by the violent muscular contraction of epilepsy or electric shock. The head of the humerus is jammed behind the glenoid surface and is in full medial rotation (Figure 3.3). There may

be indentation of the front of the head of the humerus.

The radiographic appearances are all too easily and all too often passed as normal but the following appearances are suggestive:

1. The head of the humerus and the glenoid cavity may overlap in the anteroposterior view; this can happen with a normal shoulder if the view is slightly oblique. The presence of a gap between these bones rules out dislocation.
2. The cortex of the head of the humerus appears to be an irregular but complete circle (Figure 3.4a). This is because the head is in full medial rotation with the result that the central ray is directed along arrow L rather than arrow A (Figure 3.4b) and the head overlaps the tuberosities.

The error is facilitated by the fact that the external deformity of the shoulder is less obvious than with anterior dislocation and the limb lies in a natural posture so that, unless it is seen and felt that there is flattening in front and prominence behind, the condition may be mistaken for frozen shoulder.

Recurrent dislocation. Both anterior and posterior dislocation can recur. This is much more likely to follow dislocation in adolescent or early adult life when the greater force required to disjoint the shoulder is more damaging than what suffices in older persons. Fractures of the head of the humerus or of the rim of the glenoid surface may or may not be present, but the essential lesion is unhealed detachment of the capsule from the anteroinferior sector of the glenoid surface.

Inferior dislocation is a variant of anterior but much less frequent. Less frequent still is luxatio erecta, in which the arm sticks straight up in the air and the lateral surface of the humerus faces the glenoid cavity. It is the result of extreme abduction.

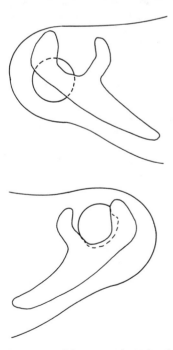

Figure 3.3. Diagram to show the alteration of outline caused by posterior dislocation of the left shoulder, as seen from above

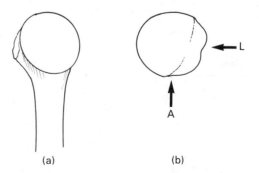

Figure 3.4. The effect of medial rotation on the radiological appearance of the head of the humerus in an anteroposterior view of the shoulder

The clavicle and its joints

The injuring force is usually generated by a heavy fall on to the point of the shoulder such as occurs in Rugby football or judo.

Acromioclavicular joint

A downward force applied to the acromion process of the scapula (Figure 3.5) can displace it downwards from the clavicle, aided by the inclination of the acromioclavicular joint. If only the acromioclavicular ligaments are torn, the costoclavicular ligaments cause the outer end of the clavicle to come to rest behind rather than above the acromion process (Figure 3.6). There is consequently not much visible deformity, in contrast to the obvious step that occurs when the coracoclavicular ligaments have been torn and allow the scapula to slide downwards and forwards. Although it is often stated that the clavicle is pulled up by the trapezius and the sternomastoid muscles, this is not so: their influence is balanced by that of the pectoralis major and deltoid, which latter is torn by the displacement. The clavicle remains in its natural position and the obvious step at the acromioclavicular joint is corrected when the shoulder is braced back and the scapula also rises.

The structure of this joint does not lend itself to successful repair of the ligaments unless the joint is temporarily transfixed. On the other hand, active use from the beginning can restore satisfactory function.

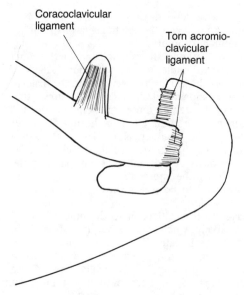

Figure 3.6. Overriding of the clavicle on the acromion process when the coracoclavicular ligament remains intact

Sternoclavicular joint

Dislocation usually results from a blow on the point of the shoulder that drives the medial end of the clavicle forwards (Figure 3.7, 2a) so that it forms a prominent bulge in front of the first costosternal joint. Although it can be replaced by voluntary retraction of the shoulder, the joint is

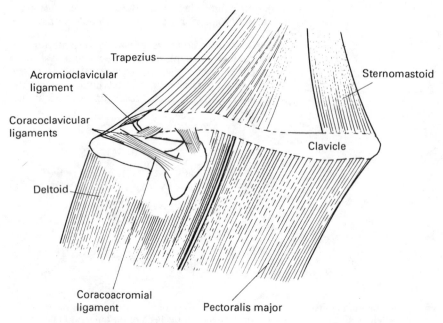

Figure 3.5. The acromioclavicular joint

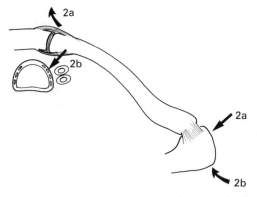

Figure 3.7. The forces that damage the sternoclavicular joint cause the clavicle to rotate slightly about a vertical axis; 2a drives the lateral end of the clavicle backwards and 2b drives it forwards as well as inwards

unstable and repair is unlikely to be successful. Persistent displacement does not usually cause more than inconvenience, although the deformity may be objectionable to a woman.

Much rarer is posterior dislocation (Figure 3.7, 2b). Although the displaced inner end of the clavicle may press upon the trachea or the great vessels in the base of the neck, it is easily replaced by retracting the shoulder and pulling the clavicle forwards by hand. The anterior sternoclavicular ligament remains in continuity and once the clavicle is back in place it stays there.

Fracture of the clavicle

This usually follows a fall on to the outstretched hand. In children the fracture is often of the greenstick variety but, as in adults, it may be widely displaced. The weight of the limb pulls the lateral fragment downwards but although a spike on the medial fragment can be very prominent under the skin, it very rarely punctures it. Most fractures occur near the middle of the bone; the few that occur at one or the other end have effects similar to acromioclavicular and sternoclavicular dislocations but they have the advantage that they heal by bone and without deformity if they are fixed surgically.

Fracture of the humerus

Fracture of the head is most often the result of direct impact and may be accompanied by fracture of the glenoid surface or by dislocation of the shoulder.

Fracture of the neck of the humerus occurs much more often and usually because of a fall on to the hand. In children, the most familiar result is to produce what appears to be an adduction fracture-separation of the epiphysis of the head, of the type 2 of Salter and Harris (1963). In fact, if a lateral radiographic view is available, it shows that the distal fragment has moved forwards as well as proximally in relation to the head. The direction of the force along the bone tends to encourage this displacement. Occasionally, the displacement of the distal fragment is sufficient to embed it in the deltoid muscle, from which an operation may be required to release it. Another reason for operating is that the tendon of the long head of the biceps is caught in the fracture.

The displacing forces can often be counteracted by pulling on the arm while it is flexed and abducted at the shoulder but this is an awkward posture to maintain for a fortnight or so while the fracture becomes sticky. Internal fixation can be used to maintain correction but in a child the remodelling that occurs with growth is such that all but the most severe deformity can be overcome.

In old persons, the deformity is often one of abduction at the fracture, which is because the anatomical neck of the humerus weakens with age, particularly where it has lost the attachment of the muscles of the rotator cuff.

Fracture of the neck of the humerus sometimes accompanies anterior dislocation of the shoulder. If there is sufficient soft tissue connecting the fragments it may be possible to replace them, but if the fragments are completely separate the shaft of the bone may come to lie by the trunk while the head remains dislocated and has to be operated on.

Injuries of the soft tissues

The structures at risk are shown in Figure 3.8. Although injuries of the separate anatomical structures have been distinguished by such terms as subdeltoid bursitis, adhesive bursitis and frozen shoulder, rupture of the supraspinatus and bicipital tendinitis, it is not realistic to consider the structures separately and, when referring to lesions of the rotator cuff, it must be remembered that more than this musculotendinous structure is involved. Moseley's term, superohumeral joint, has much to commend it.

Superohumeral joint

In young persons the structures are tough enough to resist rupture by wrenches and are more likely to be injured by impact. A fall on to the outstretched hand can drive the head of the humerus against the arch of the acromion and coracoid processes of the scapula and the ligaments between them. The upper part of the rotator cuff

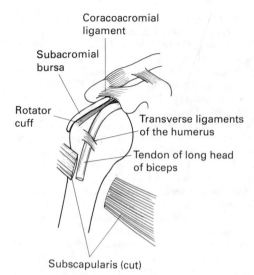

Figure 3.8. The rotator cuff and related structures

(Figures 3.2, 3.8) is bruised and swollen and may be partly ruptured; there is an effusion into the subdeltoid bursa and perhaps into the synovial sheath of the tendon of the long head of biceps. Movements of the joint are hampered by pain and, once the swelling has subsided, there may be adhesions in and around the bursa, but there is usually full recovery of function.

The supraspinatus is only part of the rotator cuff of four muscles (Figure 3.2) but it is the most vulnerable part, particularly after middle age. The tendon of insertion receives its blood supply from the muscle medially and the humerus laterally but, as the years pass, the tendon between these two sources of supply becomes less well nourished, weaker and to some extent worn away. At this stage, either a wrench or impact can tear the tendon more or less completely and more or less extensively. The smaller tears can recover fairly well but without good physiotherapy there is likely to be persistent pain, stiffness and weakness. Massive avulsion of the cuff renders the shoulder almost powerless because, without the stabilizing influence of the rotator cuff on the head of the humerus, the other muscles acting on it lose their mechanical advantage.

There are two rare sequels of injury in younger persons. The first is rupture of the rotator cuff that leaves a hole into which the head of the humerus can slip in certain positions of the joint. The victim feels something 'give', a slip or a jerk while lifting the arm at the shoulder and either allows the limb to drop or checks the movement of elevation, which may then be completed. The condition can be likened to a pothole in the road: if a wheel misses it, movement is smooth and unimpeded, whereas if the wheel passes over it,

movement is at least checked abruptly.

The second condition results from thickening and redundancy of the subdeltoid bursa. During abduction of the shoulder the bursa becomes crumpled up against the coracoacromial arch and movement is impeded, but it can usually be completed, with a click or a jerk, by adjusting the position of the shoulder.

Tendon of the long head of the biceps

Occasionally, rupture of the transverse ligament of the humerus allows this tendon to slip out of its groove, but the other damage that is likely to accompany this lesion makes it of little clinical importance. Rupture of the tendon is a well-known feature of the degeneration of age but it has little lasting effect on the use of the limb. When the muscle contracts it causes a characteristic ball-like lump to form below the deltoid muscle, with a noticeable hollow above it.

Rupture of muscles

Rupture of most of the muscles around the shoulder has been recorded at one time or another as a result of violent effort or forcible wrenching, but a heavy crushing force applied to the front of the shoulder can transect the pectoralis major. The resulting gap quickly fills with blood but it can still be felt; there may be marks of impact and when the muscle is contracted it forms a lump below the clavicle.

The most severe example of rupture of muscles is avulsion of the fore quarter, which is fortunately very rare, but in spite of the extent of the injury there may be very little bleeding and it has been known for a victim to walk for help, carrying the detached limb.

Wounds

The mobility of the shoulder and its numerous layers of soft tissues means that the track of a penetrating wound is likely to be obliterated when the posture of the limb is changed. This must be borne in mind when the wound is explored. Another consequence of the differential mobility of the soft tissues is the fact that the neurovascular bundle can be pushed aside undamaged, particularly by a blunt penetrating object.

Injuries of the brachial plexus

Because the plexus spans the angle between the spine and the axilla it is vulnerable to forces that drive the head and the shoulder apart, as can happen in road accidents and during birth (Figure 3.9). Depending on the amount of force and the

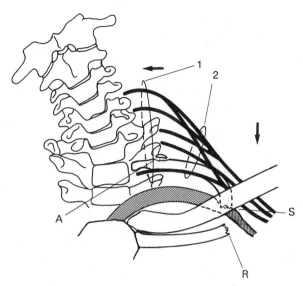

Figure 3.9 The effect of violent separation of the head and the shoulder by the forces shown by the arrows: A, avulsion fracture of the first rib; R, fracture of the first rib by the clavicle; S, crushed segment of the subclavian artery between the clavicle and the first rib; 1, site of avulsion of nerve roots from the spinal cord; 2, approximate site of tearing within the plexus

speed at which it is applied, the effect on the brachial plexus ranges from partial tearing of the upper trunk to avulsion of the entire plexus from the spinal cord. Mild tears in the substance of the plexus result in frayed ends of nerves that may not be pulled apart. Although when such a case is explored the lesion appears to be in continuity, spontaneous recovery is not to be expected except in neurones that have been stretched and have suffered no more than axonotmesis, which coexists with neurotmesis when the plexus has not been completely torn.

When roots are torn from the spinal cord, their sheaths come to form saccular extensions of the subarachnoid space that are well shown by myelography. Whether or not Horner's syndrome occurs depends on whether or not the first thoracic root has been torn.

There are often marks of injury on the side of the head and on the shoulder concerned; when these are found in an unconscious person, there should be immediate suspicion of injury to the brachial plexus. There may also be avulsion fracture of the tubercle of the first rib on the injured side. Less often, the lower roots are injured by traction with the arm above the head, as may happen during road accidents and birth (Klumpke's paralysis).

Costoclavicular compression

Forcible depression of the shoulder girdle may not only injure the brachial plexus but may also crush the subclavian artery between the clavicle and the first rib and may break the latter, and perhaps others lower down.

Reference

Salter, R. B. and Harris, W. R. (1963) Injuries involving the epiphyseal plate. *Journal of Bone and Joint Surgery*, **45A**, 587

4

The arm and elbow

Arm

Fractures and dislocations

The humerus is the first long bone that has so far been considered and it will be used as a model for fractures of long bones in general. Most are broken by bending or a sharp blow or twisting, but pulling and pushing forces are sometimes responsible. Each has its characteristic pattern, although this may be altered by secondary injuring forces, by gravity or by muscular action. The characteristic patterns of fracture are shown in Figure 4.1, but their essential simplicity may be modified by irregularities of structure.

Fracture by bending

When a beam is loaded as in Figure 4.2, it undergoes deflection, which is shown with exag-geration in Figure 4.2b. The concave surface of the beam is in compression and the convex surface is in tension; somewhere in between, shown dotted, there is neither compression nor tension. If the beam fails, tension will break it straight across as far as the neutral line, beyond which compression causes it to shear in one or both directions (Figures 4.1a, 4.2b). The wedge-shaped fragment that results is correctly known as a shear piece, which is more informative and more accurate than the more popular (and attractive) term butterfly fragment. Although it often happens that the fracture line deviates from transverse in one direction only, or appears to be a simple oblique one, it may be recognizable that there is a fine crack, such as is shown by the dotted line in Figure 4.1a. This is of practical importance because careless manipulation, whether open or closed, can create a separate shear piece and may complicate treatment.

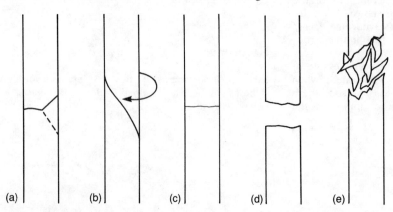

Figure 4.1. Patterns of fracture caused by (a) bending; (b) twisting; (c) tapping; (d) pulling; (e) pushing

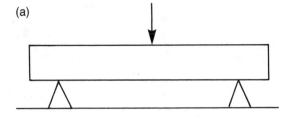

(a)

(b)

Figure 4.2. Fracture by bending

Fracture by bending can result from either a blow or a fall on to the hand. In the case of a blow, if this is delivered while the arm is at the side, sufficient energy can be transmitted to the trunk to break one or more ribs or injure adjacent structures such as the diaphragm, liver or spleen.

Fracture by twisting

Spiral fractures of the shaft of the humerus mostly result from falls on to the hand but the role of torque is most obvious in fractures caused by arm-wrestling. Once a spiral fracture has occurred, secondary forces can cause a second fracture (Figure 4.3).

Fracture by tapping

Tapping is used to denote a sharp blow with little or no follow-through. It causes a simple transverse crack (Figure 4.1c). Although it is often described as being undisplaced, even a crack is evidence of displacement, however slight.

Fracture by pulling

Avulsion fractures are characteristically transverse (Figure 4.1d). When they are caused by violent muscular action the fragments are pulled apart and may remain so, but if the energy is generated from without, secondary forces can cause overlapping, tilting and twisting.

Fracture by pushing

Bursting or compression fractures (Figure 4.1e) are comminuted and shortened. Overlapping may be the result of either impaction or mere shortening by muscular action; the distinction is easily made clinically.

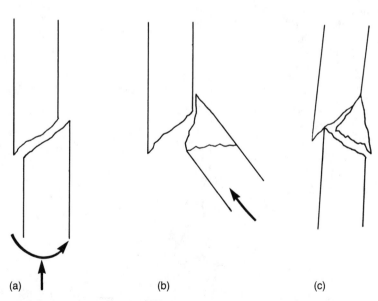

(a)   (b)   (c)

Figure 4.3. a, Torque applied in the course of a fall causes a spiral fracture; b, longitudinal compression, perhaps combined with torque or bending may then cause a second fracture, after which (c) gravity and muscular tone may restore approximately normal alignment but with more or less offset and shortening

Fractures of the shaft of the humerus

Spiral fractures are among the easiest of all fractures to treat because non-union is almost unknown, even though abduction of the proximal fragment sometimes causes wide separation. The functional effects of such malunion are much reduced by the freedom of movement of the shoulder joint. It is remarkable that, in spite of its close relationship to nearly one-third of the shaft and its possible tethering where it passes through the lateral intermuscular septum, the radial nerve is so rarely injured by fractures here.

Transverse fractures can create much more difficult conditions for union because the fragments have fairly small ends with a high proportion of cortical to cancellous bone and are easily distracted by gravity and by injudicious attempts at splinting, such as a hanging cast. Apart from adding to the weight of the limb below the elbow, a hanging cast often extends little or no distance above the fracture, which consequently receives no support as well as being distracted.

Fractures of the lower end of the humerus

The patterns of fractures in adults are shown in Figure 4.4.

Low spiral fractures (1) and transcondylar fractures (2) follow falls on to the hand, respectively with and without torque applied to the humerus.

Intercondylar fractures (3) can follow a fall on to the point of the elbow, which drives the blunt wedge in the trochlear notch of the ulna into the corresponding groove in the humerus. In this case there is usually evidence of injury over the point of the elbow.

T- and Y-fractures (4) might be caused in the same way but they can also result from hyperextension. The tip of the olecranon process is driven forcibly into the olecranon fossa of the humerus and the tough anterior capsule is rendered fully taut, thereby jamming the radius and ulna hard against the humerus and forming a couple with the olecranon.

Fracture of the capitulum (5) is one of the rarest and most interesting of this group of fractures. It occurs after middle life and how it occurs may be inferred from the disposition of the marks of injury, as seen in the course of exploring the elbow joint. The cartilage of the head of the radius shows shredding and tearing in an arc that is directed proximally in the line of the humerus when the forearm is pronated, as it would be during a fall on to the hand. Such marks of injury would occur if the head of the radius were to slip beneath the capitulum; this would make the ligaments of the elbow taut and if they did not rupture they would force the radius hard against the capitulum and so split off its front part. The signs of damage on the main and loose fragments of the humerus are consistent with this (Figure 4.5). It is of only theoretical interest to speculate on the balance between the strengths of, respectively, the bone and the ligaments and between the magnitude of the force and the speed of its application.

If there is more than slight displacement, these five fractures do not respond well to closed manipulation.

The patterns of fractures in children are shown in Figure 4.6.

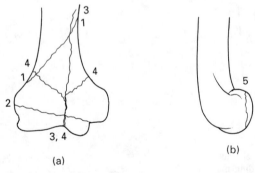

(a)

(b)

Figure 4.4. Fractures of the lower end of the humerus in adults (details in text)

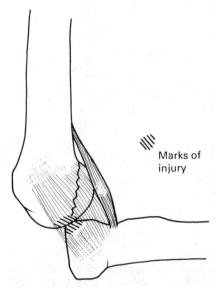

Marks of injury

Figure 4.5. Posteroinferior subluxation of the head of the radius

Supracondylar fracture of the humerus

(1, Figure 4.6) is the most important fracture in this region because of its serious complications and because of the difficulty of achieving and maintaining a good position after more than slight displacement of a fracture has occurred. In this connection, some misconceptions exist.

The injury is caused by a fall on to the hand and the direction of the force follows the line of the radius. There is thus a bending force applied to the lower end of the humerus and there may be an element of rotation because the radius is on its lateral side.

If the lower fragment is not driven right off the upper one it is rotated and it is tilted upwards on the lateral side, whereas if it is completely displaced it lies behind the upper one; it is not rotated and it is tilted little or not at all (Figure 4.7). In the lateral radiographic view corresponding to Figure 4.7a there is often a lateral view of one fragment and an oblique view of the other, but there may be oblique views of both. In the lateral view corresponding to Figure 4.7b there is a lateral view of each fragment.

According to the amount of displacement at the moment of injury there is more or less damage to the brachialis muscle and more or less risk of damage to the median nerve and the brachial artery. The medial corner of the proximal fragment may bruise the skin from the inside but only rarely does it pierce it.

It is well known that the brachial artery can be damaged by the proximal fragment of the humerus and that what may appear to be mere bruising of the artery is in fact the outward sign of tearing of the intima and perhaps thrombosis, for which surgical repair is required. It is less well known that the brachial artery can be kinked by traction on the supratrochlear artery because it has been pulled back by the medial corner of the distal fragment (Rowell, 1975). Figure 4.8 shows how this artery is tethered as it participates in the anastomosis around the joint.

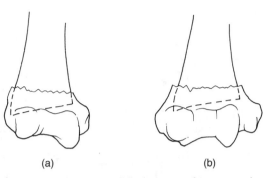

(a) (b)

Figure 4.7. The nature of displacement of a supracondylar fracture of the humerus as seen from behind: a, rotation and tilting of the lower fragment; b, complete backward displacement of the lower fragment

Rarely, the lower end of the humerus is displaced medially and this can cause the tendon of the biceps brachii to be drawn between the fragments (Figure 4.9).

Only rarely is the ulnar nerve injured.

Manipulation. A clear understanding of these matters helps one to appreciate the difficulty of dealing successfully by closed methods with severely displaced supracondylar fractures. However, that is not to say that such understanding guarantees success because although one may achieve a good position of the fracture it may be impossible to maintain it. Among the aids to keeping the fragments in place that have been recommended are, first, keeping the forearm pronated so as to reduce the pull of the muscles on the medial side of the lower fragment; secondly, placing the elbow in extension; thirdly, flexing the elbow as much as possible so as to lock the fragments together by the tension in the posterior hinge of soft tissues. The first two methods are worth trying but the third is misguided because a taut hinge will not lock an oblique fracture in place.

Various methods of manipulation have been recommended but rarely with sufficient detail to make them clear. In principle, one should reverse the forces that caused the displacement. This can be done by gripping, for example, the right arm with one's left hand so that the thumb can be placed behind the lower fragment. The right hand grips the forearm (Figure 4.10) and pulls on it while the left steadies the arm and the left thumb pushes the lower fragment forwards. It may be helpful to have the elbow at an angle of about 120 degrees to start with and then, after pulling and pushing as has been described, to flex it as far as possible without affecting the colour of the hand. It can be very dangerous to the median nerve and the brachial artery to hyperextend the elbow before pulling on the forearm.

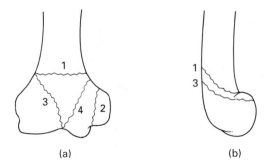

(a) (b)

Figure 4.6. Fractures of the lower end of the humerus in children

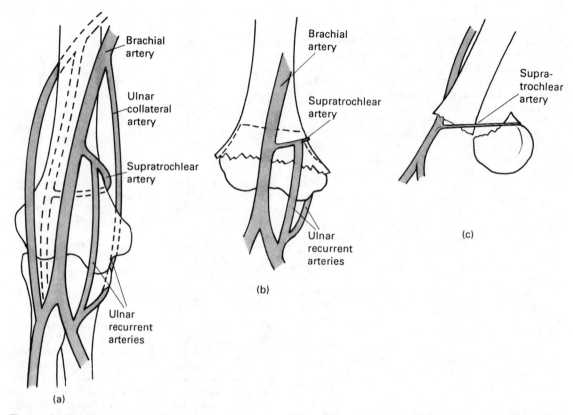

Figure 4.8. Kinking of the brachial artery by the supratrochlear artery: a, the vascular anastomoses; b, c, the effects of displacement on the supratrochlear artery

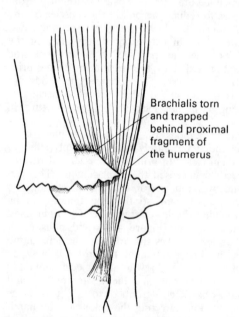

Figure 4.9. Partial tearing of the brachialis muscle and trapping of the tendon of the biceps brachii by the broken end of the humerus after supracondylar fracture

Once the elbow is flexed as far as it will safely go (usually to about 50 or 60 degrees) it is kept so with the aid of the right hand while the right thumb is placed on the medial and the right forefinger on the lateral epicondyle of the humerus (Figure 4.11). One then tests the stability of the fracture by gently rocking it backwards and forwards and from side to side and also twisting it.

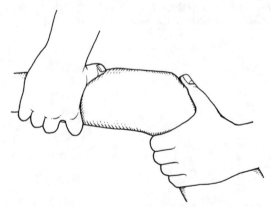

Figure 4.10. A useful grip for replacing a supracondylar fracture of the humerus, which is on the right

With the milder fractures little or no movement can be felt after a successful manipulation; with others, one recognizes that a good position is easily lost or that one is never achieved. In these cases, further manipulation should be undertaken and different positions of the elbow and of rotation of the forearm may be tried in the hope of finding a stable arrangement.

The foregoing presents manipulation as both a method of treatment and a method of diagnosis, e.g. of the stability of the fracture in a good position. If it is clear that the fracture cannot be kept in a good position, one may be content to flex the elbow as far as it will go without affecting the circulation of the hand. Again, an angle of 50 or 60 degrees is often possible. If the lower fragment lies directly behind the upper, as shown in Figure 4.7b, remodelling with growth may completely correct the deformity but if the lower fragment is tilted and twisted as in Figure 4.7a the deformity will be permanent and result in cubitus varus and the so-called gunstock deformity. This does not interfere with function but it is ugly.

Part of the difficulty in maintaining a good position with fractures of this sort arises from the fact that, however much control one may have over the forearm with plaster of Paris or any other means of external splintage, one cannot expect this to exert much control over rotation of the proximal fragment, especially when the forearm lies in medial rotation in a sling.

When operating on badly displaced supracondylar fractures of the humerus, one must remember that because the subcutaneous fat has been split or torn, the median nerve and the brachial artery may be immediately under the skin.

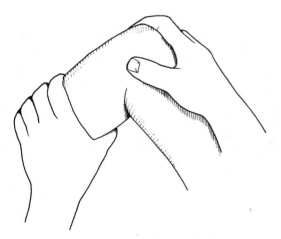

Figure 4.11. A grip for testing stability of a supracondylar fracture of the humerus, which is on the left, after manipulation

Anterior displacement of the lower fragment after supracondylar fracture is rare. In theory, one should place the elbow in full extension but in practice this is an awkward posture and it makes it difficult either to make use of the hand or to keep it elevated. Having the elbow flexed does not always lead to deformity at the fracture but when it does occur the deformity is not dangerous, it has little effect on function and it is corrected by remodelling.

Fracture of the medial epicondyle (2, Figure 4.6) can occur as an isolated injury or in combination with dislocation of the elbow. In either case, it is caused by avulsion. In spite of the proximity of the ulnar nerve this is rarely injured, but if it *is* injured it should be explored and the opportunity may be taken to replace the epicondyle and fix it in place. In the ordinary way this is not necessary and, even when the fragment is trapped in the joint, it may be possible to extract it by fully extending the wrist and fingers while the joint is dislocated or by applying gentle faradic stimulation to the flexor muscles.

Fracture-separation of the capitulum (3, Figure 4.6). McLearie and Merson (1954) showed that this injury is in effect the lateral part of a supracondylar fracture that may be combined with transient ulnohumeral dislocation. It results from a fall on to the hand. The tilting of the fragment that is seen in the more severe examples of the injury is the result of muscular action after the fracture has occurred and not because the extensor muscles pulled it off.

There are two matters of particular importance with this fracture: the first is that non-union and delayed ulnar palsy usually follow mild fractures (Jeffery, 1958); the second is that more serious displacement is generally regarded as requiring open correction.

As shown radiographically, the ossific nucleus of the capitulum is usually quite large but it is not always appreciated by the viewer that the capitulum as a whole is a good deal larger. This means that, although the fracture appears to be only slightly displaced, the fragment may be of such a size that both the radius and the ulna articulate with it (Figure 4.12) and that muscular action may gradually displace the fragment to an unacceptable extent. It is therefore important to radiograph mild fractures two or three times during the first week or two in case operation should become necessary.

It might be thought that if this injury follows a fall on to the hand the manipulation described on pages 29–30 would be successful but McLearie and Merson found that it could make matters worse.

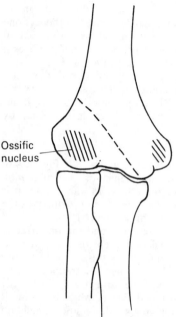

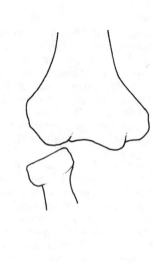

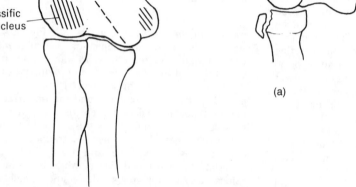

(a)

Figure 4.12. The difference between the sizes of the capitulum and its ossific nucleus

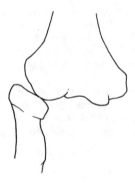

They recommended redislocating the elbow, which can be done quite gently (page 33), and then putting it back in joint. Although they succeeded in a number of successive cases, the writer has been less successful and it needs to be remembered that gradual redisplacement may still occur after a successful manipulation and one may justifiably question the propriety of the possible need for a second anaesthetic in order to fix the fracture. Although it is often stated that the fracture can be fixed by stitching the soft tissues, these are most readily available behind the fracture, where they offer no mechanical advantage. Transfixion with Kirschner's wire is more reliable.

Fractures of the medial condyle of the humerus (4, Figure 4.6) are rare because the direction of the force breaking the lower end of the humerus is almost always towards the lateral side and because the coronoid process of the ulna offers less resistance to dislocation than does the head of the radius. Accurate and reliable replacement is likely to require internal fixation.

Fractures of the radius and ulna

As with fractures of the humerus, the patterns in adults differ from those in children.

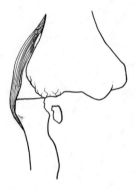

(b)

Figure 4.13. Anteroposterior view of fractures of the head and of the neck of the right radius: a, radiographic appearance; b, arrangements at the moment of injury

Fractures of the head and neck of the radius. Adults fracture the head whereas children tilt the epiphysis. When the elbow is radiographed the forearm is supinated (Figure 4.13a) whereas when a person falls forward on to the hand the forearm is pronated. If the elbow is explored it can be shown that when the forearm is pronated the depression in the head fits accurately against the capitulum, which may show corresponding signs of injury (Figure 4.13b). The size of the depressed fragment depends upon how far the head slides sideways under the capitulum. More than slight lateral displacement causes the head to strip up the attachment of the lateral ligament of the elbow to the humerus. If the elbow is kept flexed in a sling or a plaster cast while the tear is healing, the scar can prevent the movement of the ligament that is necessary for full extension of the elbow; rotation of the forearm is not affected.

Shattering of the head of the radius occurs when it is driven hard against the capitulum without sliding sideways. The victim is usually past middle age. The proximal movement of the radius that is necessary to allow this shattering to occur means that the interosseous membrane and the inferior radioulnar ligaments are torn.

Rarely, the proximal epiphysis of the radius is knocked right off rather than just tilted. It may retain a tenuous synovial stalk but even without this the epiphysis will survive in the synovial liquid; however, it usually has to be fixed in place while it heals.

Proximal end of the ulna. In adults the olecranon process is either pulled off by muscular action, which results in a transverse fracture with separation, or is comminuted by direct impact. These fractures rarely occur in children, who are more likely to show an obliquely longitudinal fracture of the olecranon. This may look so mild as to require little attention but one should be aware that it may nevertheless be accompanied by subluxation of the head of the radius that may go unrecognized. If this should happen, the subluxation can increase and lead to distortion of the epiphysis that makes correction increasingly difficult (Figure 4.14). The

injury is a mild form of Monteggia fracture-subluxation but it can have disproportionately serious consequences.

Elbow

Dislocations at the elbow

Pulled elbow. This injury occurs when a toddler's elbow is jerked sharply. The child is held by the hand and either stumbles or is pulled away from danger: a click may be heard, a cry certainly is and then the child is reluctant to use the elbow. The explanation is that the neck of a child's radius is more tapered than that of an adult and that the head can be pulled down and jammed into the annular ligament. It is easily released by quickly (usually) supinating the forearm: there is a click, a cry and the elbow is restored to use.

Dislocation of the elbow. A fall on to the hand usually drives the forearm backwards and more or less laterally off the lower end of the humerus, tearing the soft tissues mainly at the front and on the inner side of the joint. Rarely, the displacement is sufficient to result in damage to the median nerve or the brachial artery. Occasionally the forearm is displaced medially.

Usually the elbow is more or less immobile but occasionally the damage to muscles as well as ligaments is such that the elbow can be moved freely in all directions and requires surgical repair to keep it in position. This is most likely in heavy and elderly persons.

Manipulation is most easily carried out if the forearm is made to retrace its outward path but it is widespread practice to pull on it with the elbow flexed to about a right angle. This ignores the fact that at the moment of dislocation the elbow is at an angle of about 150–160 degrees and the forearm is pronated. The manoeuvre used is similar to that for supracondylar fractures (pages 29–30; Figure 4.10), but it is often necessary to adjust the angle of the elbow and the degree of pronation of the forearm until the elbow slips back into joint. This can be done very gently when the exact position of dislocation is adopted. Once the elbow is flexed even slightly above a right angle there is no risk of its dislocating again, except when the soft tissues have been badly torn, as described above.

If the medial epicondyle has been pulled off it can usually be felt as a mobile nodule on the medial side, but if it has been trapped in the joint there is a springy block to flexion at 50–60 degrees and the bare bone and the tucked-in muscles can be felt through the haematoma on the inner side (Figure 4.15).

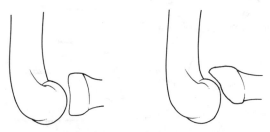

Figure 4.14. Deformation of the head of the radius as a result of altered distribution of pressure during growth

Recurrent dislocation of the elbow. This rare condition occurs mostly in children. By the time that the patient seeks attention, repeated displacement may have so reduced the size of the coronoid process of the ulna as to suggest that this is the cause of the trouble and numerous ways of augmenting it by bone, muscle or ligament have been described. In fact, as Osborne (1963) showed, the deficiency is in the extensor muscles and the lateral ligament and if this is repaired dislocation ceases. Why this deficiency should persist does not appear to have been explained.

Fracture-dislocations of the elbow

General comminution. Great violence can shatter any or all three bones and their repair can make heavy demands on the surgeon's skill.

Monteggia's injuries (Figure 4.16). The anterior and posterior patterns of injury are well known, the lateral less so. The anterior injury can result from violent and excessive pronation of the forearm whereby the radius is levered out of joint with both the ulna and the humerus and at the same time breaks the ulna, which has provided a fulcrum. In other cases the account of the injury suggests that it is a variety of dislocation of the elbow in which the ulna stays in joint above but breaks lower down. If the ulna breaks through the

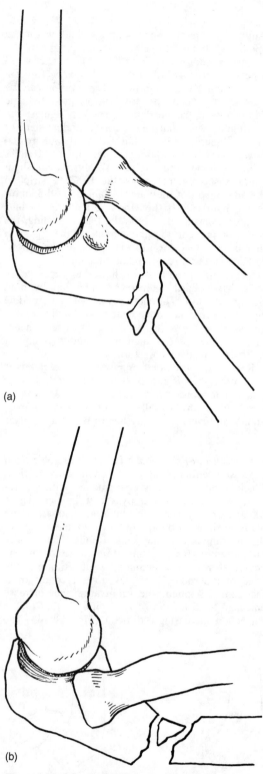

(a)

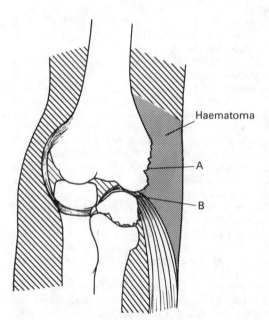

Figure 4.15. The palpable characteristics of a trapped medial epicondyle of the humerus: A, raw bone felt through the haematoma; B, the flexor muscles turning sharply into the joint

Haematoma

A

B

(b)

Figure 4.16. Monteggia's fracture-dislocations: a, anterior; b, posterior; c, lateral

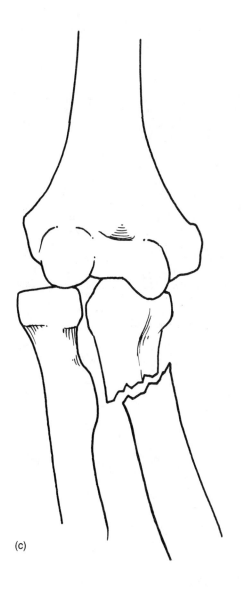

(c)

happen, the lateral side of the joint should be explored in case the annular ligament has got in the way. In children, particularly with greenstick fractures, holding the forearm in full supination in a long plaster cast is usually sufficient to maintain the proper shape of the ulna but occasionally the proximal end of the ulna is cocked up so much that it becomes embedded in the flexor muscles and has to be released surgically. In this case it is wise to fix the fracture of the ulna. In adults it is almost always necessary to fix the ulna. If, as sometimes happens with the posterior injury, the head of the radius is broken, this may safely be removed once the ulna has been fixed.

Soft tissues

The damage that results from fractures and dislocations needs no further consideration.

Flaying

When a rubber-tyred wheel passes over a limb lying on a hard surface the tyre drags the skin beneath it, tearing it from its deep attachments and sometimes splitting it as well so that it becomes a sheet with more or less attachment at one or both ends. The muscles may be separated from each other and perhaps torn from bone; fractures and fracture-dislocations sometimes occur. Even when the skin remains intact it has been more or less severely and extensively crushed and its viability can be further reduced by being distended by a massive haematoma; it may not be easy to decide how best to treat it.

Avulsion of the biceps

This occurs typically in men past middle life who make a sudden effort such as lifting a heavy weight. It is much more disabling than rupture of the tendon of the long head of the muscle because it puts the whole muscle out of action. It should be repaired, which needs to take account of the fact that the tendon is not a simple cord-like structure attached to the tuberosity of the radius but has quite an extensive 'tail' that has to be wrapped partway round the bone.

Brachial artery

The two main causes of injury are crushing and tearing, which are often combined when the artery is stretched over the sharp edge of the proximal fragment of the humerus. Complete division leaves no doubt about the diagnosis but crushing can cause confusion and lead to misguided treatment that can have disastrous consequences.

trochlea the result is the rare anterior fracture-dislocation. The posterior Monteggia injury is more obviously related to posterior dislocation of the elbow.

The lateral pattern of injury is rare but it is important because it can occur in a sufficiently mild form in children for the injury to be mistaken for an oblique fracture of the ulna, the displacement of the head of the radius being unperceived (page 33). Severe injuries of the lateral sort can interpose the humerus between the proximal ends of the radius and ulna.

The key to successful treatment is to restore the natural shape of the ulna; this will almost always replace the head of the radius. Should this fail to

A bruised segment of artery may have pulsation both above and below it but still be blocked. This happens when the intima is torn in such a way that it forms a flap that blocks the lumen or because it sets off local thrombosis. Pulsation distal to such a lesion is the result of good collateral circulation and it may be questioned whether anything needs to be done to relieve the obstruction. In other cases, the artery distal to the bruised segment is narrow and does not pulsate. This has been regarded as spasm, and efforts to overcome it by means of locally applied drugs, by distending the artery by injecting into it or by sympathetic blockade, have distracted attention from the cause of the narrowing, which is lack of filling. Like a balloon, an artery collapses if it is not distended by contents at a suitable pressure. The narrowing of the artery will be overcome by dealing surgically with the obstruction. This is not to say that spasm of arteries does not occur, as a result of stretching or an irritant injection, for example, but to emphasize that a narrow artery beyond a bruised segment demands that the segment be explored. A diagnosis of spasm and the use of drugs is a dangerous substitute for useful activity.

Ulnar and median nerves

When these are injured at the elbow the lesion is nearly always a combination of mainly axonotmesis with some neurapraxia and recovery is usually good, especially in children.

Reference

McLearie, M. and Merson, R. D. (1954) Injuries to the lateral condyle epiphysis of the humerus in children. *Journal of Bone and Joint Surgery*, **36B**, 84

Jeffery, C. C. (1958) Non-union of the epiphysis of the lateral condyle of the humerus. *Journal of Bone and Joint Surgery*, **40B**, 396

Osborne, G. V. (1963) Recurrent dislocation of the elbow joint. *Journal of Bone and Joint Surgery*, **45B**, 614

Rowell, P. J. (1975) Arterial occlusion in juvenile humeral supracondylar fracture. *Injury*, **6**, 254

5

The forearm

Fractures of both bones

The characteristic patterns of fractures of the radius and ulna are best shown by greenstick fractures because they allow the bones to remain in the positions of primary deformity, whereas when the bones are broken right through, gravity and muscles produce secondary displacement.

A fall forwards on to the hand applies a force that has a dorsally directed component that can reasonably be likened to extension (Figure 5.1).

Sometimes both bones are broken at the same level and are bent to the same angles (Figure 5.1a). This can be regarded as the result of a pure extension force, but more often the radius is broken at a higher level than the ulna and is bent more sharply. This adds a component of supination to the extension (Figure 5.1b) and is the most frequent pattern of fracture in the forearm; Colles's fracture is the most familiar example. Occasionally the twisting component is one of pronation (Figure 1c). Much less often the injuring force

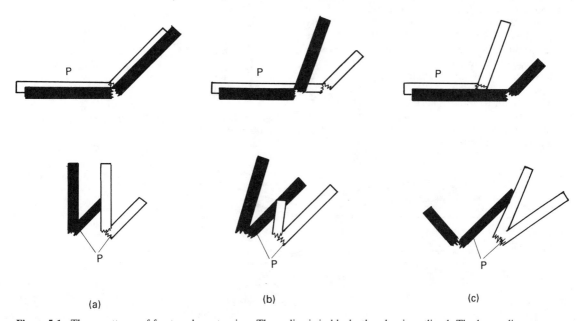

(a) (b) (c)

Figure 5.1. Three patterns of fracture by extension. The radius is in black, the ulna is outlined. The lower diagrams represent the bones seen end on. a, Extension; b, extension with supination; c, extension with pronation; P, proximal fragments

produces flexion, with or without pronation or supination; Smith's fracture is an example of this pattern.

When there is a greenstick fracture of one or both bones the deformity is easily corrected by applying a flexing and, usually, a pronating force at the fracture. This force must be maintained by suitable moulding of a well-padded plaster of Paris cast (Figure 5.2) or the deformity will recur. It is still taught by some that the remedy is to complete the fracture by breaking the hinge of bone but to do this is to deprive oneself of the guiding influence of the hinge.

In children, if the bones are broken right through and are overlapped there are often hinges of soft tissues, but before the fragments can be brought end to end it may be necessary to increase the deformity (Figure 5.3). This applies particularly to simple transverse fractures. If there is a hinge of soft tissue, simple traction cannot succeed because the hinge becomes taut before the fragments come edge to edge (Figure 5.3a). Re-creating the original deformity allows the periosteum to resume its rightful place on the proximal fragment (Figure 5.3b). It may be added that the amount of extension (or flexion in some cases) required is no more than that caused by the injuring force.

Spiral, oblique and comminuted fractures can usually be pulled out to length but, particularly in adults, they may not remain there without surgical fixation.

Most fractures of one or both bones in children are in the distal half of the forearm and if the plaster cast is moulded skilfully it is not necessary to put the elbow in plaster. There is, however, one mild-looking fracture in children that requires special care. It is little more than a crack through the radius, roughly at the junction of the upper two-thirds. There is often a slight forward bow that may not seem to require correction but it needs to be understood that this fracture occurs between supinating muscles attached to the proximal fragment and pronating muscles attached to the distal

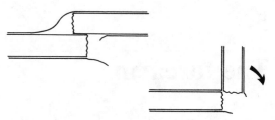

Figure 5.3. The influence of the hinge of soft tissues on an overlapped transverse fracture

fragment (Figure 5.4). Unless the fragments are locked firmly together by keeping the forearm fully pronated by including the elbow joint in the plaster cast, and so rendering the dorsal hinge taut, the muscles can considerably increase the

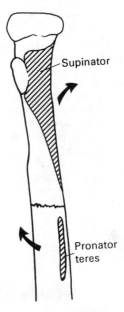

Figure 5.4. Muscles that produce deformity of a fairly high fracture of the radius

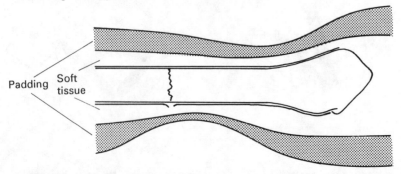

Figure 5.2. Moulding that holds the fractures in place by keeping their hinges taut. Thick padding leaves plenty of room for swelling and the indentations are offset

bowing of the radius; this deformity is not much affected as growth takes place and it can prevent full pronation.

Fractures of the radius

Galleazzi's fracture

This is familiar as a fracture of the radius a few inches above the wrist with disruption of the inferior radioulnar joint that makes it impossible to control the distal fragment of the radius except by surgical fixation. If one regards the injury as being essentially a fracture of the radius with inferior radioulnar dislocation, this definition includes fractures at the ends of the radius as well as in its shaft (Figure 5.5).

Fracture of the head of the radius

When the head of the radius is shattered by a fall on to the hand this happens because the whole bone has been displaced proximally far enough to be torn loose from the lower end of the ulna. The patient's complaints usually refer to the elbow only, but an experienced doctor will recognize in radiographs that the stump of the radius is up

against the capitulum and will seek swelling and tenderness at the wrist, where the dislocation can be shown radiographically (Figure 5.5).

Fracture of the lower end of the radius

The more severely displaced fractures of Colles and Smith will often disconnect the radius from the ulna, so rendering these notoriously unstable injuries even less amenable to manipulation and plaster. An extreme example of this type of injury occurs when the head of the ulna bursts through the skin.

If success is to be achieved in the treatment of Colles's and Smith's fractures by manipulation and plaster of Paris, the breaking forces must be reversed and the plaster must be moulded so as to maintain, respectively, either flexion with pronation or extension with supination at the fracture. However successful one's efforts may be at first, serious deformity is likely to recur; as a result, the fragments return to a position of stability with considerable deformity and the fracture quickly becomes firm. When this happens, the cast can often be removed after as little as 2 or 3 weeks, which helps to reduce stiffness of the wrist.

In the case of Colles's fracture it is still believed by some that flexing the wrist helps to prevent recurrence of the deformity, but this can be true only if flexion is sufficient to render the dorsal part of the capsule taut and consequently capable of pulling on the distal fragment(s). More than slight flexion of the wrist restricts the use of the hand and the full flexion that would theoretically be necessary is not an acceptable posture for a matter of some weeks.

A rare variant of Colles's fracture occurs in young persons; it includes avulsion of the styloid process of the ulna and disruption of the radioulnar joint. The small piece of bone can burst through the soft tissues, which then come together and prevent it from returning to its bed when the radius is manipulated. This in turn prevents the lower end of the radius from being restored to its rightful position (Figure 5.6). Unless this 'valvular' lesion is recognized and corrected surgically the inferior radioulnar joint will suffer lasting damage.

Barton's fracture

This can be regarded as an incomplete form of Smith's fracture. It might be thought that extending the wrist fully would draw the palmar fragment into place by means of the capsule but this is not so because, as the capsule becomes taut, the carpus bears on the fragment and there is no means whereby it can be prevented from slipping proximally (Figure 5.7). Surgical fixation is required.

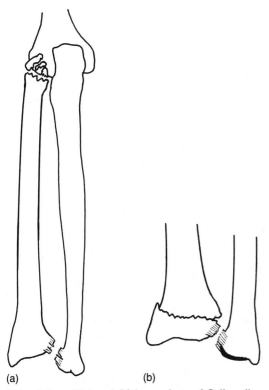

(a) (b)

Figure 5.5. a, High and (b) low variants of Galleazzi's injury

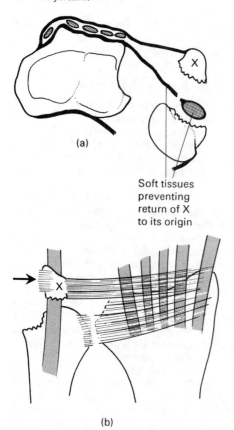

(a)

Soft tissues
preventing
return of X
to its origin

(b)

Figure 5.6. Inferior radioulnar fracture-dislocation with 'valvular' displacement of part of the ulna. (a) Transverse section at level of arrow in (b) (dorsal view)

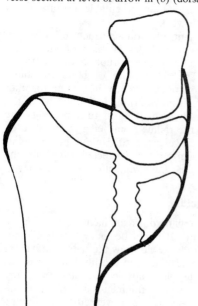

Figure 5.7. Barton's fracture

Fracture of the styloid process of the radius

This is the result of impact by the scaphoid bone and is considered in more detail in Chapter 6 (page 45).

Fracture of the dorsal edge of the radius

This fracture occurs in younger rather than older adults and is comminuted. It is the result of impact against the edge rather than against the main articular surface of the radius and it can be regarded as an abortive form of dorsal fracture-dislocation.

Fractures of the ulna

Isolated fractures of the ulna are often the result of a blow, as when the hand is raised either to strike or to protect the face. Such fractures range from a crack to comminution and considerable displacement of the fragments. Even with the mild fractures, muscular action can cause sufficient movement to delay and sometimes to prevent union of a bone that has small ends with a high proportion of relatively avascular cortical to cancellous bone. If the fracture is oblique or spiral there is less likelihood of delay in union.

Dislocations at the wrist

Radiocarpal dislocation

This is almost always a fracture-dislocation although the fracture(s) may be of no more than the very tips of the styloid processes.

Inferior radioulnar dislocation

When this occurs without fracture it is likely to be in the elderly, who have weak ligaments. It is usually unstable. Lesser injuries include detachment of the intra-articular disc by excessive rotation of the forearm; this causes clicking and weakness, which are relieved by removing the disc. Persistent and troublesome dislocation of this joint can be treated successfully by removing the lower end of the ulna but if this is merely prominent, removing a segment of the ulna is equally successful. It may be asked how much of the ulna should be removed. In the former case it is sufficient to remove only enough (about three-quarters of an inch; ≈19 mm) to enable the ulna to be clear of the radius but the stump can also be bevelled. Removing more than that can leave the stump of the ulna uncomfortably mobile among the adjacent tendons. If a segment of the ulna is to be removed a gap of ≈19 mm is sufficient.

It is worth mentioning that the relative lengths of the normal radius and ulna vary greatly (Figure 5.8). The naturally long ulna can be distinguished from relative lengthening after fracture of the radius by the presence of facets on both the ulna and the triquetral bone (Figure 5.8b).

Injuries of soft tissues with fractures

Injuries of muscles

More or less damage to the soft tissues inevitably accompanies fractures. This damage may be inflicted directly by the force that breaks the bone and results in tearing or crushing in the area of impact or it may result from indirect injury, as when a fall on to the hand displaces the broken bone and so damages the soft tissues around it. If muscles are torn across by the broken ends of the bones, this may occur where the nerve and blood supply enter the muscle as a neurovascular bundle, termed by Brash (1955) a neurovascular hilum. Such damage may thereby separate the main bulk of the muscle from its nerve and blood supply. If this happens there is no advantage – and there may be dangers – in preserving the dead muscle. The tendons can be attached to suitable motors but it is remarkable how much function can be retained by a much-reduced amount of muscle. In the forearm, for example, the whole of the flexor digitorum superficialis can be removed without

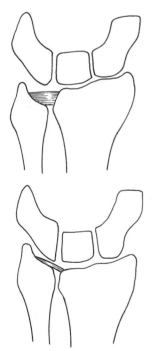

Figure 5.8. Natural variations in the length of the ulna

serious loss of function, provided that the flexor profundus is working normally.

As the muscles' bellies give way increasingly to tough and slippery tendons in the distal part of the forearm, the ends of the bones make their way to the surface between them rather than through them, with the result that even marked displacement may do remarkably little damage to the soft tissues in the area.

Injuries of tendons

Occasionally, the tendon of extensor pollicis longus ruptures 2–8 weeks after Colles's fracture. The fracture affects the bed of the tendon but the writer's experience has been that such a fracture has always been very mild, with only a small step in the bone. Although rupture by attrition has been offered as an explanation, this seems unlikely with such a mild fracture and it may be that a combination of damage by impact and ischaemia following bleeding into an almost intact and unyielding sheath plays a part. A personal study of nearly 100 mild fractures of this sort showed that delayed rupture was rare even among these and also that there was no clinical means of predicting its occurrence.

Occasionally, the tendons crossing the lower part of the radius become trapped there and require surgical withdrawal.

Injuries of nerves

In spite of the severe deformity that occurs with some Colles's fractures, injury of either the median or the ulnar nerve is exceptional. Occasionally, however, the carpal tunnel syndrome develops later because of fibrosis around the nerve.

Injuries of soft tissue without fracture

Avulsion

Fingers are sometimes torn off with their tendons and muscles; less severe injuries leave the part attached although muscles have been torn. One piece of evidence that this has happened is that one or more tendons visible in a wound take a less than normally direct course and may sag noticeably. Even when a muscle belly has been torn right through, this may not be evident until its sheath has been opened and it is found that what appeared to be bruising is in fact a haematoma between, and infiltrating, the torn ends of the muscle belly.

Flaying

There is nothing to add to the account of this type of injury that was given in Chapter 4 (page 35).

Deep wounds

These are usually in the distal part of the forearm, on the flexor surface, and they are most often the result of putting the hand through glass; occasionally they follow assault and, rarely, attempted suicide. The forearm may be cut to the bone but, even with less severe injuries, the less-experienced surgeon's greatest difficulty is likely to be the correct identification of the divided structures. To this end, the following recommendations should be borne in mind:

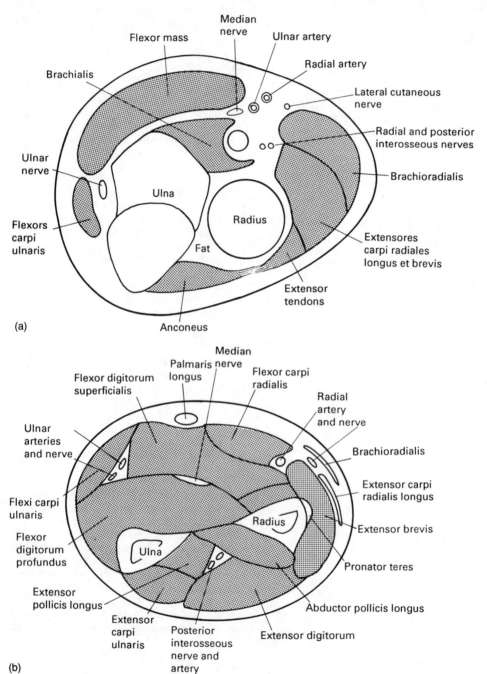

Figure 5.9. Cross-sectional diagrams of the forearm: a, near the elbow; b, in the middle of the forearm; c, near the wrist

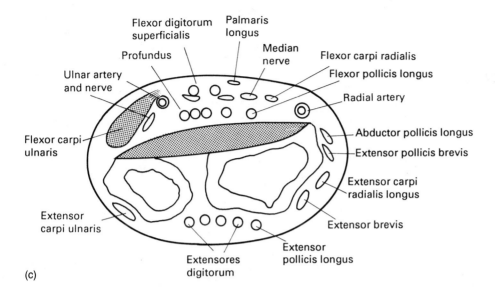

(c)

1. Have available a cross-sectional diagram of the forearm at the level of injury (Figure 5.9).
2. Have the fingers exposed so that the results of pulling on the stumps of muscles or tendons can be observed.
3. Use a tourniquet, at least while identifying the structures.
4. Any divided structure can retract, whether up a well-defined sheath or along the bed of loose connective tissue in which it normally lies. Sometimes an artery or a nerve projects from one surface; this usually means that the other end has retracted. Experience teaches, first, that any retracting structure is likely to leave at least traces of blood behind it and, secondly, that when the tissues have been cleanly cut the less they are disturbed by dissection the easier it is to use their natural relationships to identify them. The temptation is to start dissecting the visible structures but it is often possible to find retracted structures by the careful use of retractors, a good light and fine forceps while the tissues are otherwise undisturbed. 'Milking' and posture can also be helpful.

Reference

Brash, J. C. (1955) *Neurovascular Hila of Limb Muscles*, E. & S. Livingstone, Ltd, Edinburgh and London

6

The carpus

Functional anatomy

The studies of MacConaill (1941) and Gilford *et al*. (1943) threw valuable light on how the carpus works. They can be summarized as regarding it as a clamp that can be loosened and tightened and also as a chain, the links of which are the radius, the lunate and the capitate bones, with a peculiar role for the scaphoid.

The clamp

Extension of the wrist tightens the ligaments and jams the bones firmly together in the close-packed position. For those that are not familiar with this term, it can be compared with the different-sized contents of a container that has been shaken for some time. When the container is shaken, the level of the objects in it gradually falls to a level that then remains constant, no matter for how long the shaking continues. This is because the shaking causes the smallest objects to work their way to the bottom and the largest to the top, with those of intermediate size arranged accordingly. Arranged in this way, the contents occupy the smallest possible volume and are said to be close-packed.

The chain

During extension the capitate bone tilts on the lunate and that tilts on the radius; the scaphoid follows suit. During flexion the tilts are reversed (Figure 6.1). Sideways movements of the wrist are centred near the head of the capitate bone, which rotates in its lunate cup and takes the other bones of the carpus with it. The scaphoid bone takes part in these movements by twisting slightly around a

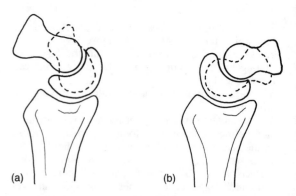

Figure 6.1. The carpal chain: a, extension; b, flexion. The scaphoid bone has the broken outline

roughly longitudinal axis and rotating rather more about a roughly transverse axis. The result is that during radial deviation the bone tilts forwards and looks short and broad, whereas in ulnar deviation it looks tall and slim (Figure 6.2). This change in outline can be likened to that of a man making a courtly bow, in which his trunk twists a little and bends more. In this way the scaphoid bone can follow the movements of both rows of the carpus; it can be likened to a person standing with a foot on each of two moving horses: all is well for as long as the movements of the horses are properly coordinated.

Patterns of injury

Figures 6.3, 6.4 and 6.7–6.13 show the main patterns of injury of the carpus, which can be

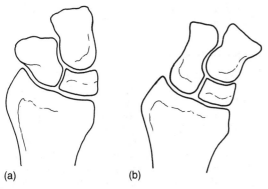

Figure 6.2. The effect of (a) radial and (b) ulnar deviation of the wrist on the apparent shape of the scaphoid bone as seen in anteroposterior radiographs

placed in two groups: that in which the fractures are no more than cracks and chips (Figures 6.3, 6.4a) and those in which displacements are obvious although their precise nature can be difficult to distinguish among the numerous and overlapping shadows in radiographs (Figures 6.4b, 6.7–6.13). For all the variety and visual complexity of some of the injuries, they are capable of explanation in the light of the functional anatomy of the

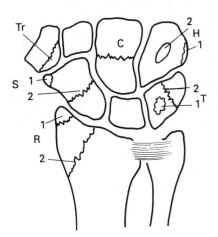

Figure 6.3. Cracks and chips in the carpus: C, capitate; H, hamate; R, radius; S, scaphoid; T, triquetral; Tr, trapezium

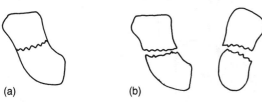

Figure 6.4. Fractures of the scaphoid bone: a, anteroposterior view of a crack; b, anteroposterior and lateral views of a fracture with separation

wrist, in which the concepts of close-packing and links are fundamental.

Cracks and chips results from a fall on to the hand when the wrist is close-packed and most of the disruptive injuries occur when it is loose.

Cracks and chips

A fall on to the hand can be regarded as concentrating much of the force into the head of the capitate bone so that it acts as a hammer, with the radius as an anvil. Although the head of the capitate looks well rounded in both anteroposterior and lateral views of the wrist, the separate bone shows quite a well-marked angle between the proximal and the radial aspects of its head.

In Figure 6.3, H1, R1 and S1 are generally regarded as sprain-fractures but it may be questioned whether this is the case with S1. First, the ligaments attached to the tuberosity of the scaphoid bone are tough and extensive; secondly, the writer's examination of a large number of radiographs yielded a series of fractures that are represented by Figure 6.5. The depression of the distal fragment shown by fracture (d) suggests that it may have resulted from impact by the trapezium and trapezoid bones, which have more than slight mobility on the distal articular surface of the scaphoid bone, and some radiographic appearances have suggested that the radial edge of the trapezium had been driven into the scaphoid and had split off part of the tuberosity.

The most frequent fracture in the carpus is a dorsal chip fracture of the triquetral bone, T1 in Figure 6.3. Although generally regarded as a sprain-fracture, it follows a fall on to the hand and is more likely to have been chipped or pinched off by contact with a neighbour during forcible extension. Fractures of the body of the bone (Figure 6.3, T2) are rare and are the result of force transmitted towards the ulnar side by the head of the capitate bone. Force transmitted towards the radial side either cracks the waist of the scaphoid bone (Figure 6.3, S2) or is transmitted through the

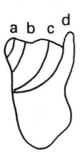

Figure 6.5. Fractures of the distal end of the scaphoid bone

bone and breaks off the styloid process of the radius (R2), which may also be displaced. These three fractures can be regarded as being of the tapping sort (Chapter 4, page 26), which is consistent with the fact that they run at approximately right angles to the long axes of the bones. It is worth mentioning that although the cartilage on the scaphoid bone may remain intact, these harmless-looking fractures sometimes proceed to non-union.

Fractures of the body of the trapezium (Figure 6.3, Tr) are rare and are probably the result of impact or crushing.

Fractures of the neck of the capitate bone (Figure 6.3, C) are also rare and it is not certain whether they are caused by a tapping or a bending force.

Fracture of the hook of the hamate bone (Figure 6.3, H2) is the result of direct violence and it may be accompanied by damage to the deep branch of the ulnar nerve, which crosses it.

Fractures of the scaphoid bone

Many are mere cracks (Figures 6.3, S2; 6.4a) but others show displacement in two or more views (Figure 6.4b). Some of these may be caused by forcible extension, when the dorsal edges of the radius and the trapezium come close together and act as a joint fulcrum, which is aided in its effect by the strength of the palmar part of the capsule. In other cases the scaphoid bone suffers the fate of the standing horseman whose steeds part company.

If the bones of the carpus are not close-packed, the carpal chain can become buckled instead of flexing and extending as a whole (Figure 6.6). When this happens the scaphoid bone is unable to conform with the opposite movements of its neighbours and is broken by bending, in which the dorsal edge of the radius plays a part, rather than by tapping. In such cases it may be noted that the

radiological gap between the scaphoid and the lunate bones is wider than usual.

Scapholunate diastasis

The scapholunate joint is normally no more than ≈3 mm wide. Separation of the two bones is bound to occur if the lunate is dislocated; it can also accompany fractures of the styloid process of the radius when the scaphoid bone is displaced with the styloid process and is thereby torn from the lunate bone. Separation can occur without fracture, in which case its existence is liable to be overlooked and its consequences misinterpreted. After a fall on to the hand, the patient complains of pain in the wrist, which is found to be swollen and tender in the anatomical snuffbox. This is taken to be evidence that there is a fracture of the scaphoid bone even though none is shown radiographically. The symptoms persist, radiography is repeated and a plaster cast is reapplied, perhaps several times. Swelling and tenderness in the snuffbox are signs of an effusion into the carpus but not all effusions come from a broken scaphoid bone: some come from tearing of the scapholunate ligament. Occasionally the widened gap is accompanied by foreshortening of the scaphoid bone, which occurs when the ligaments around the bone are torn, as well as in radial deviation (Figure 6.2).

An extreme, and very rare, form of scapholunate separation is dorsal dislocation of the scaphoid bone and the most likely explanation is that there is extreme radial deviation, which tilts the bone forwards, and that it is accompanied by supinating (S) and longitudinal (L) forces that drive its proximal pole over the dorsal edge of the radius (Figure 6.7).

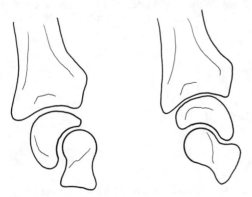

Figure 6.6. Buckling of the carpal chain

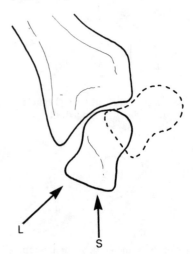

Figure 6.7. Flexion of the scaphoid bone precedes its dorsal dislocation, which is shown by the broken outline

Dislocation and fracture of the lunate bone

If the carpal chain is buckled far enough, the head of the capitate bone can escape from its lunate cup (Figure 6.6) and, having done so, it either regains its natural relationship with the radius and, as it were, kicks the lunate out of bed (Figure 6.8) or it remains behind the lunate bone, which remains in place on the radius (Figure 6.9). This is usually described as perilunate dislocation but ablunate is more accurate. In some cases the scaphoid bone is also broken and the result is transscaphoablunate fracture-dislocation (Figure 6.10). The distal components are dorsally displaced and overlap the lunate and the proximal fragment of the scaphoid bone.

A rare but interesting fracture-dislocation is one in which the head of the capitate bone has been broken off and comes to lie upside down (Figure 6.11). This can be regarded as a variety of capitolunate disruption that takes place through the neck of the capitate instead of between the two bones (Figure 6.12). Whether the head is spun round as the rest of the bone goes dorsally or as it moves back into place is a matter for speculation, not of practical importance.

Fracture of the lunate bone

This rarely occurs without dislocation and it more often appears as crumbling of a bone weakened by ischaemic necrosis (Kienböck's condition) than as a result of impact.

Severe radiocarpal disruption

Figure 6.13 shows an extreme example of radio-carpal fracture-dislocation such as would result

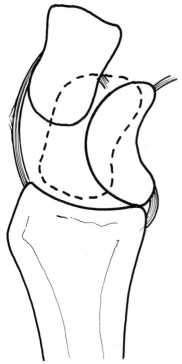

Figure 6.8. Dislocation of the lunate bone. The scaphoid bone has a broken outline

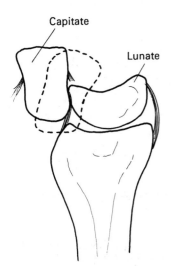

Figure 6.9. Ablunate dislocation of the carpus. The scaphoid bone has a broken outline

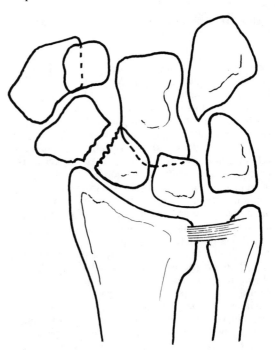

Figure 6.10. Transscaphoablunate fracture-dislocation

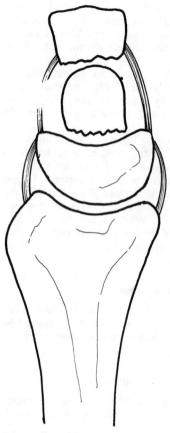

Figure 6.11. Fracture of the neck of the capitate bone with inversion of the head

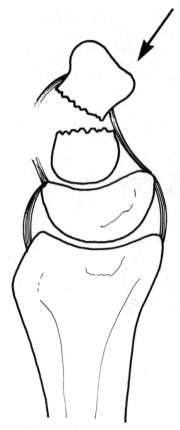

Figure 6.12. An intermediate stage of fracture of the neck of the capitate bone with inversion of its head

from violence of such degree that it drives the carpus and the styloid process off the radius, breaks the scaphoid bone and at the same time severely disrupts the carpus.

The details of these complicated disruptions of the carpus vary a good deal within the general patterns described and the variations presumably reflect differences at the moment of impact in the precise arrangements of the bones, the amount of movement that is possible between them, the amount, direction and speed of application of the disruptive force and the protective effect of muscular action. In the same way, the fragments of something that has been dropped and broken have sizes, shapes and distribution that one would not expect to be precisely reproduced if an identical object were dropped from the same height and with the same orientation in space.

Many of these injuries can be successfully manipulated with anaesthesia and various manoeuvres that aim to reverse the displacing forces have been described. Although, for example, flexing the wrist loosens the carpal clamp and might

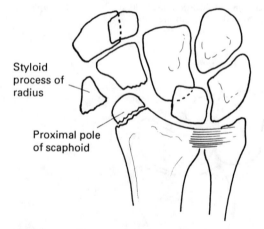

Styloid process of radius

Proximal pole of scaphoid

Figure 6.13. Transscaphoablunate fracture-dislocation with fracture of the styloid process of the radius

therefore be expected to help the displaced bones to go back into place, the most generally useful method is to pull for perhaps a minute or more on a fully relaxed limb. In many cases, however, the damage to ligaments has been such as to make surgical fixation and repair necessary if the normal arrangement of the carpus is to be restored.

References

Gilford, W. W., Bolton, R. H. and Lambrinudi, C. (1943) Mechanism of the wrist joint. *Guy's Hospital Reports, 92*, 52

MacConaill, M. A. (1941) The mechanical anatomy of the wrist joint and its bearing on some surgical problems. *Journal of Anatomy*, **75**, 166

7

The hand

Although falls on to the hand occur with great frequency the impact is almost always on to the heel of the hand, with the result that any injuries are in, or proximal to, the carpus.

Carpometacarpal joints

These are injured singly or in combination, most often by a force directed proximally along one or more of the metacarpal bones. In most cases the bases of these bones are displaced dorsally but occasionally they are displaced towards the palm. In either case, dislocation is almost always accompanied by at least chip fractures.

Bennett's fracture-subluxation

Although this is not the most frequent carpometacarpal injury it is the best known. Nevertheless, it is quite a rare injury that is sometimes overlooked or misdiagnosed because of the swelling and tenderness that are sometimes thought to be in the anatomical snuffbox.

The injury usually occurs when an ill-delivered punch is made with the head of the first metacarpal instead of the head of the third. The bone is driven proximally and at the same time it is flexed on the trapezium, from which it is displaced when the prominent ridge on the flexor surface is broken off (Figure 7.1). It will be noted that the displaced metacarpal bone causes a swelling that is distal to the anatomical snuffbox although the associated haematoma spreads superficially into its hollow. In addition, tearing of the palmar tissues at the base of the thenar eminence enables the

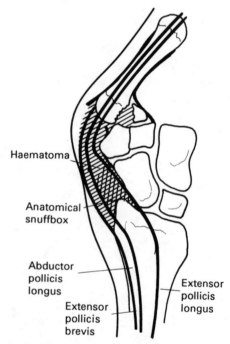

Figure 7.1. Bennett's fracture-subluxation and the resulting swelling

haematoma to spread into this but the spread into the palm is limited by the attachment of the adductor pollicis to the shaft of the third metacarpal bone (Figure 7.2). As a result, the thenar eminence is obviously larger than normal but because the blood is deep to the muscles there is no visible bruising in the palm, at least initially.

The knowledgeable observer should be able to make a confident diagnosis of a recent Bennett's

50

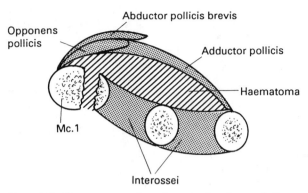

Figure 7.2. Transverse section through the base of the thenar eminence to show the spread of blood into it

injury on clinical evidence alone and may also find that by pulling gently on the thumb the lump at the distal margin of the anatomical snuffbox is abolished. After a few hours, however, the swelling spreads and as it increases makes it more difficult to recognize the lump and to locate the tenderness precisely. If the radiographer is asked to focus on the scaphoid bone the examiner's attention may be concentrated thereon; because the fracture of the metacarpal is not always clearly shown by films centred on the scaphoid bone it may be unrecognized and the injury may be incorrectly treated as a result.

Although in theory the fracture can be held in place by pressures exerted as shown in Figure 7.3a, in practice it is all too easy to misapply the pressure on the head of the metacarpal, as shown in Figure 7.3b. Even if the two pressures are applied as shown in Figure 7.3a, there is a strong tendency for the deformity to recur and the pressure required to prevent this can cause a sore at S. Various methods of splintage, with and without traction, have been devised but the most satisfactory method of treatment is to screw the fragments together. If this is done correctly, a plate adds nothing to the security of fixation.

If, as sometimes happens, the base of the metacarpal has been comminuted it may be best not to attempt any sort of correction or splintage but to encourage function from the beginning. In passing, one may suggest that for fractures into joints in general there are two methods of treatment available: one is to replace the fragments accurately, fix them securely and move the joint; the other is to accept the deformity and move the joint from the beginning. In the latter case, although the radiological appearances are alarming, function can be very good even years later, whereas malunion after several weeks of unsuccessful splintage can cause lasting stiffness and discomfort.

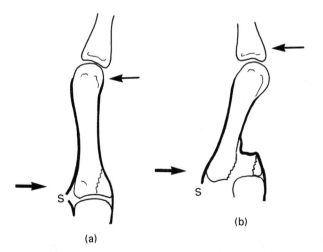

Figure 7.3. Pressure applied (a) correctly and (b) incorrectly after Bennett's injury. S, Site of possible pressure sore

Fracture-subluxation of the fifth carpometacarpal joint

This injury occurs more often than Bennett's but it receives little attention. It resembles Bennett's injury in its cause, its nature and its instability but it differs in that occasionally dislocation occurs without fracture.

Although there is an opponens digiti minimi, opposition of the little finger is very much less than that of the thumb but it does play a part in the action of cupping the palm and gripping round objects in it; its range has been known to increase strikingly and to compensate for the loss of other fingers. Even in its normally small range it is a useful movement and, unlike the thumb, there is no supplementary movement within the carpus. Derangements of the joint can have disproportionate functional effects, which make it wise to consider internal fixation when particularly fine control of the little finger is necessary. It may be fifth in number among the digits but it is by no means the least important.

Other carpometacarpal injuries

The importance of these injuries lies in the crippling effect that multiple dislocations can have and in the fact that they are liable to be overlooked until the opportunity for fully successful treatment has passed. The reasons for this are that they occur infrequently, that the hand appears swollen rather than deformed and that the radiological appearances can be confusing. An experienced doctor will find the following evidence to arouse clinical suspicion: (1) a history of considerable violence such as occurs in a motor bicycle accident; (2) the hand looks not only swollen but broad; (3) the fingers can be neither bent nor straightened fully. The metacarpus is effectively shortened and the dorsal displacement of the base(s) of the metacarpal bone(s) has the effect of shortening the extensor tendons (Figure 7.4). The hand looks broad, partly because it has been shortened and partly because it is swollen. Radiographers can unwittingly play a part in medical failure to diagnose the condition if they offer anteroposterior and oblique views of the hand. An inexperienced eye can fail to notice that the carpometacarpal joints' spaces have been replaced by overlapping shadows (Figure 7.5). An oblique view is provided because it helps to separate the shadows of the four metacarpal bones that overlap in a lateral view of the hand but it has the disadvantage that it can make the overlapping of carpal by metacarpal bones much less obvious (Figure 7.6). For this reason, it is a good general rule when there is any suspicion of fracture in the hand to request a lateral view of the suspect bones(s). An experienced radiographer will sometimes provide one even though it has not been asked for.

Dislocation of one or more of the central three metacarpal bones is very rare but much of the foregoing applies and internal fixation of these unstable injuries is usually required.

It is open to question whether these dislocations follow a blow on the knuckles(s) or a heavy blow in the palm. The history usually gives no clue and there may be no sign of impact at either of the places mentioned.

Fractures of the metacarpal bones and phalanges

Like the injuries of the carpus, these can be divided into cracks and chips and those with considerable displacement.

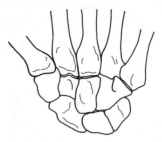

(a)

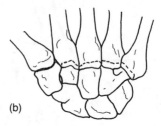

(b)

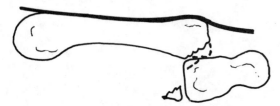

Figure 7.4. Effect of dorsal carpometacarpal dislocation on the extensor tendon. Alternative fractures of the carpal and metacarpal bones are shown dotted

Figure 7.5. a, Spaces of the carpometacarpal joints; all four may not be shown on the same film; b, overlapping of four carpometacarpal joints

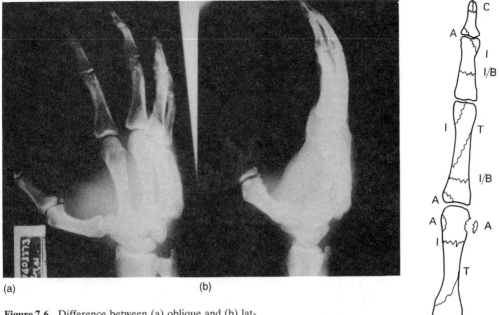

(a)   (b)

Figure 7.6. Difference between (a) oblique and (b) lateral views of dislocation of all four carpometacarpal joints

Figure 7.7. Examples of mild fractures in the hand, caused by A, avulsion; B, bending; C, crushing; I, impact; T, twisting

Cracks and chips

The fractures of these miniature long bones (Figure 7.7) are caused by the usual five forces (Chapter 4) that are applied by the various activities of work and recreation. Such fractures are stable and require no more than protection during cautious use of the hand.

Fractures with considerable displacement

The most severe injuries of this kind are often open, multiple, combined with dislocations and the result of great violence, e.g. injury by machinery or explosives. There are, however, some characteristic patterns of injury that require consideration. It should be emphasized that although many of these fractures are small in scale they are not small in importance and they should not be regarded as minor injuries.

Fractures of metacarpal bones (Figures 7.8, 7.9)

Fracture (a) in Figure 7.8 is a typical flexion fracture of the base of the first metacarpal bone that results from impact on the head. In this respect it resembles Bennett's fracture-subluxation

but the fracture is usually impacted and therefore stable and it can be treated by cautious use from the beginning.

Fracture (b) in Figure 7.8 is fairly stable in deformity, which is maintained by muscular action and is not usually prevented by plaster of Paris. The history of injury usually leaves it in doubt whether it was the result of bending or twisting associated with impact end-on.

Fracture (c) in Figure 7.8 is the well-known boxer's fracture. Whether or not it is impacted, it is stable only in deformity and the effect of even 50 or 60 degrees of deformity on function is so small that the fracture is best treated by cautious activity from the beginning. The prospect of successful treatment by even carefully moulded plaster casts is similar to that with Bennett's injury (Figure 7.3). For all its justification in theory, the most dangerous way of treating this sort of fracture is by pressure and counterpressure (Figure 7.8d) because it renders the hand useless while it is being treated, it can cause both stiffness and pressure sores and it may not prevent eventual deformity.

Fractures e and f in Figure 7.8 may not matter when only one metacarpal bone is affected and the

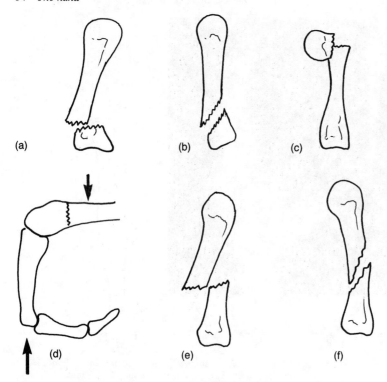

Figure 7.8. Fractures of metacarpal bones: a, lateral; b, anteroposterior views of the first; c, d, fifth; (d) shows the application of pressure and counterpressure with the finger bent; e, fracture by bending or heavy impact; f, fracture by twisting

deformity is not severe. It is not difficult to understand how a rolling fall on to the side of the hand could cause spiral fractures of the fifth and possibly the fourth and even the third metacarpal bone as well but the history usually throws no light on how a spiral fracture occurs in one of the central bones in the series.

Fracture (A) in Figure 7.9a is a simple avulsion fracture and it usually heals by bone. When the joint has been dislocated, a sprain-fracture such as this shows whether or not the ligament has been

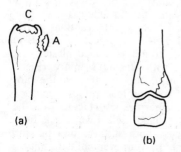

Figure 7.9. a, Avulsion (A) and compression (C) fractures of head of metacarpal bone; b, fracture of the base of the second metacarpal bone by impact

trapped in the joint and how nearly the ligament has returned to its proper position. It is therefore useful for guiding treatment.

Fracture (C) in Figure 7.9a is caused by impact, which depresses the sector of the head of the metacarpal bone that receives the blow. The fracture is wholly within the joint, with the result that even though it is in a good position the bony part loses its blood supply, dies and later crumbles.

Fracture (b) in Figure 7.9b is rare and occurs only at the base of the second metacarpal bone. A blow on the head of this bone causes the blunt wedge of the trapezoid to split off one prong of the base of the metacarpal.

Sometimes the styloid process at the base of the third metacarpal bone is a separate fragment, not the result of fracture.

Fractures in the fingers

Fractures of the terminal phalanges (Figure 7.10a–d)

Fracture (a) is more often caused by hyperextension than by flexion; its importance lies in the fact

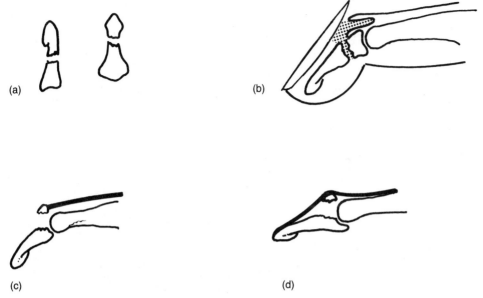

Figure 7.10. Fractures of the terminal phalanx caused by (a) flexion or extension, (b) flexion, (c) avulsion and (d) impact

that it occurs in the narrow part of the bone that is mostly, if not entirely, cortical. Union can be very slow and it sometimes fails altogether. If the nail has been lost and does not grow again the fingertip can be troublesomely unstable. Serious malunion can also occur and impair function.

Fracture (b) is sometimes overlooked. When the nail has been uprooted, the sharp flexion of the fingertip is not at the joint but at the fracture. When this is the case, the nail provides an admirable splint for the fracture as well as keeping the edges of the nailbed together; it should therefore be preserved and replaced after careful toilet of the wound beneath.

Fracture (c) is the well known, so-called mallet (finger) fracture. It is caused by avulsion and it can be difficult to treat successfully, especially when the fingertip is bent more than 30–40 degrees. When the deformity exceeds this it is because all connection between the extensor tendon and the terminal phalanx has been lost and the action of the flexor profundus is unopposed. Furthermore, because the extensor tendon retracts, all extensor action is now concentrated at the proximal interphalangeal joint and if this joint is naturally hyperextensible the so-called swan's neck deformity results.

Fracture (d) appears at first sight to be the same as 7.10c and is consequently likely to be referred to as a mallet (finger) fracture. However, if one

looks carefully at the radiograph one will see that: (1) the dorsal fragment is a block rather than a chip; (2) the gap is quite wide; (3) the fingertip does not droop, which is the characteristic feature of a mallet, or drop, finger. The dorsal swelling at the base of the nail may give the appearance of drooping of the tip but radiographs show clearly that this is not so.

A fourth feature of this not very frequent injury is that the terminal phalanx is displaced slightly in a palmar direction. If the terminal phalanx is extended, in the belief that mallet fingers, with or without fracture, should be treated in hyperextension, the subluxation becomes more obvious and this is the clue to the nature of this injury. The extensor lip is not pulled off by the tendon but is sheared off by a combination of longitudinal compression and hyperextension in much the same way as the small fragment of Bennett's injury is sheared off (Figure 7.1). Figure 7.10c is incorrect because it shows the extensor tendon as being attached to the extensor lip of the phalanx whereas in fact its attachment extends well down the bone and is stripped up and not torn across (Figure 7.10d). Once the nature of the injury has been recognized it can easily be shown that the fingertip can be extended against resistance (McMinn, 1981).

Fractures of the middle and proximal phalanges (Figure 7.11a–c)

Fracture (A) in Figure 7.11a is caused by avulsion. Many such heal by bone but if the gap is

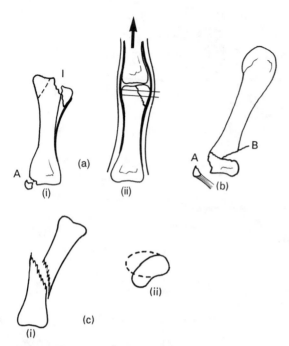

Figure 7.11. Fractures of the middle and proximal phalanges: a, caused by avulsion (A) or impact (I) before (i) and after (ii) fixation; b, caused by avulsion (A) or bending (B); see also Figure 7.8e; c, spiral fracture. The dorsal view (i) shows little displacement but the end-on view (ii) shows obvious rotation

more than a few millimetres wide and the fragment is tilted so that the two broken surfaces no longer face each other, surgical repair may be necessary in order to prevent persistent laxity of the joint. One useful result of this fracture is that it shows whether or not the ligament has been tucked into the joint, as sometimes happens.

Fracture (I) in Figure 7.11a results from asymmetrical impact by the phalanx distal to it. Symmetrical impact may shear off both condyles (shown dotted). Unlike a crack fracture in the same place, this is unstable and requires surgical fixation. In this connection, it should be remembered that a lateral exposure of the condyle can result in a good deal of damage to the collateral ligament and consequent stiffness. This can be avoided if it is possible to pass one or two fine wires across the fracture after it has been replaced by suitable traction and without opening it (Figure 7.11a(ii)).

Fracture (A) in Figure 7.11b. The fragment is attached to the palmar ligament (volar plate) of the joint and often results from dorsal dislocation. It is not always recognizable in radiographs made while the joint is dislocated and it may show up

only after it has been replaced. It is therefore advisable to radiograph dislocated fingers both before and after they have been manipulated. If the gap remains wide in spite of moderate flexion of the joint after the dislocation has been corrected, one should consider exploring it, bearing in mind the fact that the fibrous sheath of the tendon will have been torn and that this will add to the scarring that will occur in the tendon's tunnel.

Fracture (B) in Figure 7.11b is caused by hyperextension and usually occurs at the base of the proximal phalanx. Although the action of the extensor apparatus has been blamed for the ease with which the deformity recurs after manipulation, a more likely explanation is either crushing or the depression of a piece of the dorsal part of the cortex, as shown. Either would leave a dorsal defect in the bone. For this reason, fixing the fracture in flexion, which does not control the proximal fragment, may not maintain a good position. It should be understood that this is a notable example of a fracture that needs a lateral view if the true deformity is to be shown.

Fracture (C) in Figure 7.11c is caused by twisting; the deformity shown radiographically (Figure 7.11c(i)) may not give rise to concern but one must remember that the distal fragment may have been twisted (Figure 7.11c(ii)) as well as slightly tilted. If the twisting goes uncorrected, when the finger is flexed with its neighbours it will be seen to lie across one of them.

Fractures (e) and (f) in Figure 7.8 (see page 54) can occur in phalanges as well as in metacarpal bones and no more needs to be said about them.

Dislocations of the digits

Brief references to these have been made in connection with some of the sprain-fractures but dislocation as such deserves attention. This section deals also with injuries of ligaments without persisting displacement.

Most interphalangeal and metacarpophalangeal dislocations have the distal component displaced dorsally and in some cases laterally as well.

The painful, swollen digit that has been injured

Usually the dislocation is present when the patient comes to hospital but sometimes there is apparently no more than pain and swelling of a joint, with a history of injury to it. The thumb is peculiarly liable to injuries of this sort. In such cases two tests are required:

1. The wobble test, in which the examiner tries to bend the suspect part from side to side in order to test its stability; this can usually be done successfully without anaesthesia.
2. Radiography; even a tiny chip can be very informative and sometimes quite a serious fracture is revealed.

Metacarpophalangeal joint of the thumb

This is subject to both acute and chronic injuries.

The chronic injury is known as gamekeeper's thumb because wringing the necks of game stresses the ulnar collateral ligament and over the years causes considerable laxity of it.

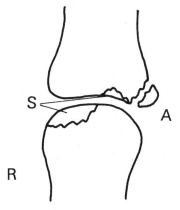

Figure 7.12. Fractures associated with rupture of the ulnar collateral ligament of the thumb: A, avulsion; S, shearing fractures; R, radial side

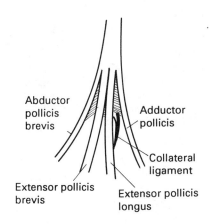

(a)

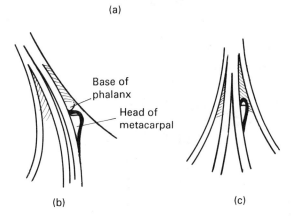

(b)   (c)

Figure 7.13. Dorsal views of rupture of the ulnar collateral ligament of the right thumb: a, the lesion is hidden by the extensor hood; b, the lesion is revealed by abduction of the phalanx; c, the torn ligament bunched up by the extensor hood

Acute rupture of the ulnar collateral ligament is the result of sudden radially directed force by a fall, kick, impact by machinery, the handlebar of a bicycle or in the course of a struggle. After the injury the thumb returns to its natural position. There is at first little swelling and no bruising but the site of rupture is tender, the wobble test is positive and there is sometimes a chip fracture, which, as Stener (1963) has shown, may be pulled off the base of the phalanx (Figure 7.12(A)) or sheared off either this bone or the head of the metacarpal (Figure 7.12(S)). When such an injury is explored the lesion may at first be hidden by the extensor hood; only when the phalanx is pulled sideways does the hood slide away to show that the collateral ligament has been torn from either the phalanx or the metacarpal bone (Figure 7.13a, b). In other cases, the torn ligament is seen to be bunched up at the proximal edge of the extensor hood (Figure 7.13c) and sometimes it is tucked into the joint.

It must be remembered that the ulnar collateral ligament is not a simple band but part of a complex structure that includes the palmar plate and that this must be taken into account, particularly when repairing a distal rupture (Figure 7.14).

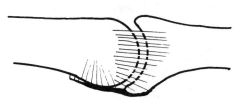

Figure 7.14. Ulnar collateral ligaments of the metacarpophalangeal joint of the thumb

Acute rupture of the radial collateral ligament is very rare, less easy to diagnose and less disabling because few natural uses of the thumb have to resist ulnar deviation at this joint.

Fixed dislocation. In one variety the phalanx is displaced dorsally and to the radial side and stays there. This is attributed to so-called buttonholing of the capsule, but when the lesion is explored it is found that the neck of the metacarpal bone is tightly gripped, not by a split in the capsule but between the tendon of the flexor pollicis longus and the tendons joining the ulnar sides of the extensor hood and the base of the phalanx. This is an example of a 'valvular' dislocation and when the taut structures are pulled apart the phalanx goes back into place quite easily. The ulnar collateral ligament is not always torn, in which case it is to some extent stripped from the bone.

Direct dorsal dislocation (Figure 7.15) is often amenable to manipulation, which, except in the hands of an expert, usually requires anaesthesia. Difficulty is most likely to arise if the palmar plate is caught between the bones (Figure 7.15(1)). It must be remembered that the existing extension deformity usually has to be increased before the phalanx can be replaced. At least part of each collateral ligament often remains intact so that the joint retains lateral stability after manipulation.

Other joints in the hand

The dislocations are similar to those in the thumb but most of them do not need to be operated on. Exceptions are those in which there are widely displaced and rotated sprain-fractures and those in which the joint is asymmetrical after manipulation. The difference from normal may be slight but it should not escape the questing eye; it means that the ligament has been caught in the joint. In other cases, although there is obvious lateral instability, the capsule has been pulled off, as a cap might be, but returns to its rightful place and will heal there if protected and have little lasting effect on function.

Palmar dislocations

These are much rarer than dorsal ones and, particularly at the proximal interphalangeal joints, are likely to cause rupture of the extensor tendon; there may also be chip fractures.

Locking finger

There are numerous causes but only one is likely to be the result of recent injury, as when a split in the collateral ligament of a metacarpophalangeal joint allows the tubercle on the side of the head of the metacarpal to slip and jam between the two parts of the ligament. This happens when the joint is flexed (Figure 7.16b). The flexor tendons are strong enough to do this but the extensor tendons are incapable of overcoming the obstruction, which can be accomplished with the other hand and is accompanied by an audible snap.

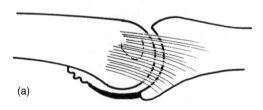

(a)

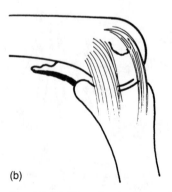

(b)

Figure 7.16. The tubercle on the side of the head of a metacarpal bone (a) becomes jammed in a split in the ligament when the joint is flexed (b)

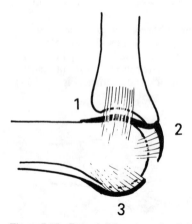

Figure 7.15. Dorsal dislocation of a digit. The palmar plate may be in position 1, 2 or 3

Injuries of tendons

Although most of these accompany wounds, some important closed injuries occur.

Wounds of tendons

Any wound over or near the course of a tendon may injure it and if a tendon is visible in a wound it cannot be declared to have escaped injury unless it has been seen to move through its full range; this is because, for example, when a flexor tendon is partly divided while the finger is flexed, the site of damage will move into the distal part of the sheath if the finger is examined in extension, as it usually is. The range of movement and the posture of the digit are unaffected by partial division of any of its tendons, whereas complete division will affect both posture and movement, even posture under anaesthesia and with full relaxation. In the case of a conscious and uncooperative child this may be difficult to recognize but the discreet use of a pin or a needle usually enables an experienced examiner to decide whether or not motor and sensory function are normal in a suspect digit.

Puncture wounds caused by small sharp objects, particularly cats' teeth and thorns, can implant bacteria in sheaths of flexor tendons or in a joint.

Closed injuries of tendons

Avulsion

Mallet finger (page 55) needs no further consideration.

A torn middle slip of the extensor digiti muscle is usually recognized too late to allow simple repair. At first the joint is swollen and painful but it can be actively extended, it does not wobble when tested and only rarely is there a fracture. With the passage of time, however, the now loosened lateral slips of the tendon separate, slide forwards and eventually come to lie on the flexor side of the axis of movement of the joint. They then supplement flexor power at the proximal interphalangeal joint and extensor power at the distal one.

Avulsion of the flexor digitorum profundus is rare and follows forcible opposition to the strongly contracted muscle, such as happens when no more than a fingertip catches the clothing in an attempt to tackle a Rugby footballer. The tendon may spring back as far as the palm, where it forms a tender lump, particularly if a flake of bone is pulled off the terminal phalanx.

Its extensive attachment to the middle phalanx makes avulsion of the flexor superficialis even less likely than that of the flexor profundus.

Rupture of tendons

In the hand the usual cause is degeneration, particularly by rheumatoid disease, which is not further considered here.

Dislocation of extensor tendons

This is most familar as a result of rheumatoid disease, which weakens and slackens the extensor hood, but it can follow a blow on or by the knuckle that displaces the tendon, usually to the ulnar side, and in so doing splits the extensor hood. When the metacarpophalangeal joint is straight the extensor tendon is in its proper place but when it is flexed the tendon slips sideways off the head of the metacarpal. If, as may happen, active extension of the flexed joint is lost, a variety of locking finger occurs.

Injuries of nerves

The only closed injury that is worthy of note is that of the deep branch of the ulnar nerve where it passes over the hook of the hamate bone. Damage can occur when the hand is used as a hammer or if a blow, by the end of a handlebar, for example, strikes this place. The lesion is rare and is easily overlooked because feeling is unaffected and the interosseous muscles may not be examined with sufficient care and forethought.

In the case of open injuries, as with tendons, diagnosis depends on suspicious awareness of the possible significance of small wounds, careful clinical examination and, ultimately, exploration. It should, however, be mentioned that if the cut ends of a nerve remain in contact, impulses can continue to cross the site of injury until the axons distal to it begin to degenerate after two or three days (Lynch and Quinlan, 1986).

Wounds

Penetrating injuries

Puncture wounds

No more needs to be said about these than that no structure in the hand is more than about half an inch ($\approx$13 mm) from the surface and that a punch in the mouth that breaks the skin over a knuckle has very likely opened the joint as well; the wound must be explored with the joint flexed.

Injuries by injection

Many substances are forced through fine orifices under high pressure and can penetrate the skin. After this, the injected substance follows the nearest fascial planes or tendon sheaths, the amount injected and the extent of spread depending on the pressure, which can range from hundreds to thousands of pounds per square inch. The damaging effects result from the irritant nature of the substance injected, whether or not the degree of tension resulting causes ischaemic death of the tissues and the fact that unless the injected substance solidifies it cannot all be removed.

Gunshot wounds

These are rare and can be very destructive. To some extent the metacarpal bones can offer protection to the tendons and neurovascular bundles, especially when small projectiles such as shot enter the back of the hand. A particularly interesting fact is the way in which the tough and slippery tendons can protect the neurovascular bundles from similar projectiles entering the side of the

palm. Being fixed, the first bones in the path of clustered shot may be shattered whereas the tendons can move away from the projectiles, taking the neurovascular bundles with them (Figure 7.17). Individual shot are more likely to move past tendons than to lodge in them.

Injury by explosion

The effects of explosion are characteristically untidy, severe and destructive. As with gunshot wounds, tendons may be less severely affected than other tissues but they offer no protection to them.

Amputation and avulsion
Amputation

Most amputations affect the fingertips and when they are carried out cleanly, whether through or

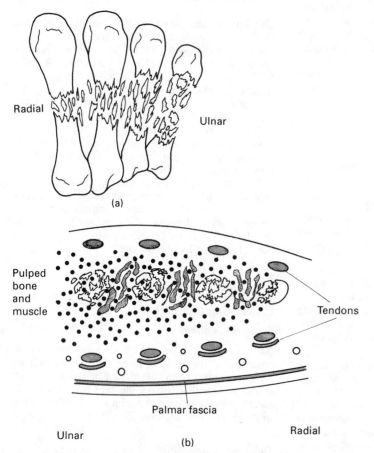

Figure 7.17. Shotgun wounds of the hand: a, diminishing damage caused by shot entering the ulnar side of the hand; b, displacement of the flexor tendons by the shot and the protection they afford the nerves and blood vessels

beyond the terminal phalanx, the soft tissues retract very little. Amputations through the middle
and proximal phalanges often leave the bone projecting but when the amputation is 'tidy' the skin
can usually be sewn together after little or no
trimming of the phalanx. 'Untidy' amputations
anywhere in the hand in which traction has played
a part do not allow this simple repair.

Avulsion

Perhaps the best-known injury of this kind is
caused when a ring catches on a projection and is
dragged forcibly off the finger. Most of the skin is
taken with it, perhaps with some bone but even
when some skin remains attached proximally the
combination of crushing and stretching makes it
unlikely that there will be any useful survival of
the sleeve of skin.

Another sort of avulsion injury occurs when the
fingers are torn off with more or less skin from the
rest of the hand and with their tendons. Because
in young persons rupture occurs more easily
through muscle than through tendon, part of the
muscle comes away with the tendon.

Flaying

These injuries are caused by machinery rather than
by rubber tyres. The planes of cleavage are between the skin and the extensor tendons on the
dorsum of the hand and either superficial or deep
to the palmar fascia. In the latter case, the neurovascular bundles and the tendons may suffer little
or no damage. Generally speaking, palmar skin
withstands these injuries better than does dorsal.

Crushing and extrusion of muscle

Crushing of the hand as a whole can be severely
destructive but sometimes the injury is confined to
the first interosseous space. The lesion appears to
be a split in the skin of the first web with muscle
sticking out of it. Such muscle has been sheared
off the metacarpal bones and has thereby been

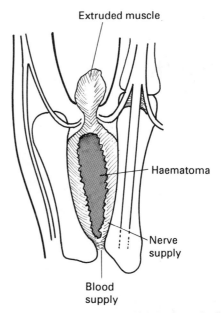

Figure 7.18. Effect of crushing between the first and
second metacarpal bones

torn from its nerve and blood supplies (Figure
7.18); it should therefore be removed. The surviv-
ing muscles of the thenar eminence can restore
useful function at the carpometacarpal joint if they
are not restrained by dense scarring in the first
interosseous space.

References

Lynch, G. and Quinlan, D. (1986) Jump function following nerve division. *British Journal of Plastic Surgery*,
39, 364

McMinn, D. J. W. (1981) Mallet fingers and fractures.
Injury, **12**, 477

Stener, B. (1963) Skeletal injuries associated with rupture of the ulnar collateral ligament of the metacarpophalangeal joint of the thumb. *Acta chirurgica scandi-
navica*, **125**, 583

8

The trunk

Chest

Fractures and dislocations

Fractures of the ribs

The first rib is sometimes broken by the muscular effort of coughing and in pregnancy both first ribs may be affected; there is little displacement. A more violent injury is caused by forcible depression of the clavicle by a heavy blow on the shoulder, which may also do damage to the subclavian artery and, rarely, the brachial plexus (Figure 3.9).

The other ribs resemble the skull in that they form a curved casing that can be broken by extensive deformation or by direct impact. Extensive deformation is the result of widespread compression and the ribs often break where they are most curved, namely at their angles; occasionally this occurs on both sides. Direct impact can break any number of ribs from one upwards. The larger the number broken, the greater the degree of deformity and the greater the degree of disturbance of the action of breathing. A single fracture shows little deformity that is the result of the blow; multiple fractures allow more or less depression of the affected part of the rib cage, which depression owes much to the blow but something to muscular action. This exerts its effect by increasing subsidence of the broken segment over the course of a few days. This effect is most striking in old persons (see page 66).

Stove-in chest is an apt term for depression of more or less of the rib cage by a blow. There are three patterns – anterior, lateral and posterior (Figures 8.1, 8.2). In the anterior variety the fractures occur on both sides of the sternum. In the lateral variety the fractures are all on one side of the chest, although it sometimes happens that both sides are injured. A particular variant may be described as a stove-in shoulder because the depressed segment lies under the scapula and follows a heavy blow on the shoulder; if it is accompanied by fracture of the clavicle there is striking deformity because the shoulder girdle subsides with part of the rib cage (Figure 8.2). The posterior variety is rare and may affect both sides.

Paradoxical respiration

This occurs when part of the chest wall moves in a direction that is the reverse of normal. The widely used term 'flail chest' is misleading because there is no resemblance to the action of a flail, which is an old tool used for threshing (Figure 8.3). The striking arm is accelerated by moving the handle and goes on moving after the handle has been brought to rest.

Paradoxical movement is in essence a sign of instability of the chest wall and in the anterior and lateral varieties of stove-in chest the movement is more or less obvious, although the inexperienced eye sometimes has difficulty in recognizing the timing of the movement, much as the inexperienced ear has difficulty in timing murmurs in the heart. When the shoulder has been stove in the paradoxical movement may be either hidden by the overhanging scapula (Figure 8.2a) or prevented by the weight of the shoulder girdle.

The rare posterior variety causes a different pattern of movement, particularly when both sides are affected. This injury virtually disconnects the rib cage from the spine and thereby deprives the muscles of respiration other than the diaphragm of

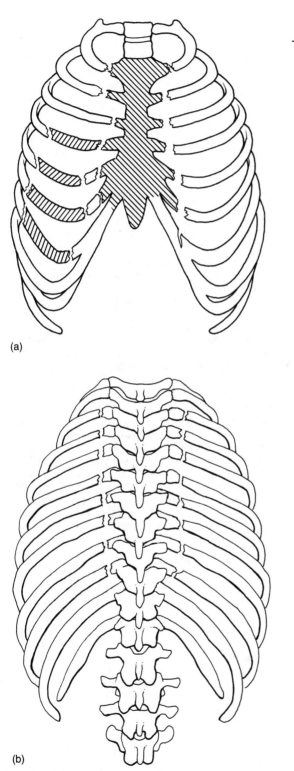

(a)

(b)

Figure 8.1. Patterns of stove-in chest: a, anterior and lateral; the shaded areas move paradoxically; b, posterior

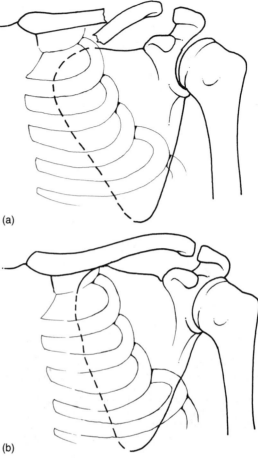

(a)

(b)

Figure 8.2. Stove-in shoulder (a) without and (b) with fracture of the clavicle

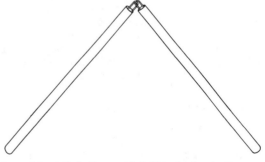

Figure 8.3. A flail. One end is held in the hands, the other does the striking

their costovertebral fulcra and renders them ineffectual, or nearly so (Figure 8.4). The diaphragm can still act and when it contracts it pulls the rib cage downwards, pushes the abdominal organs downwards and so raises the level of the abdominal wall of a recumbent person. Thus, the chest

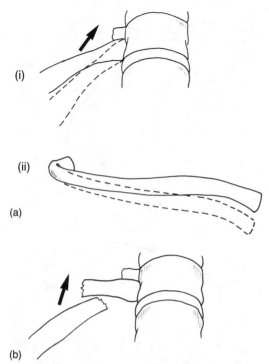

Figure 8.4. The effect of posterior fractures of the ribs on their movements during respiration. a, The muscles of respiration pull the ribs upwards and outwards on their vertebral and sternal hinges; (i) anteroposterior and (ii) lateral view of a right rib. b, After fracture of the back of a rib the normal respiratory movement is no longer possible. The arrow shows the direction in which the muscles pull

falls and the belly rises during inspiration and these movements are reversed during expiration. This can fairly be described as paradoxical thoracoabdominal movement, or more simply as seesaw paradox. It is similar to the movements that are characteristic of breathing after tetraplegia, when the diaphragm is unopposed because the other muscles of respiration are paralysed.

Fractures of the sternum

There are two varieties.

Fracture by impact. A blow on the sternum can break it across and may cause the fragments to overlap as a result of muscular action. The blow may also damage the heart. Occasionally the damage to the intercostal muscles is so extensive that the two parts of the sternum are pulled apart during inspiration as the diaphragm and the upper muscles of respiration act in opposite directions. This condition, like paradoxical movement of the sternum (Figure 8.1a), requires surgical fixation.

Fracture by bending. The sternum shows a forward bow at or near the manubriosternal junction. This is caused by a bending force applied to the spine. If this part of the chest, as seen from the side, is likened to a gothic arch it will be readily understood that if the back part of the arch is broken the front part will be broken as well (Figure 8.5). Unless this possibility is considered, the coexistence of a high fracture of thoracic vertebrae may go unsuspected; even when it is suspected, this part of the spine can be difficult to show clearly with radiographs.

Fractures of the spine

The thoracic part of the spine is much more vulnerable in its lowest levels because above them the rib cage reduces the amount of movement that is possible and thereby provides useful protection. This means that the considerable force required to cause serious damage to the spine is likely to result in damage to the spinal cord as well. Perhaps the most dangerous condition of the spine is extensive ankylosis because in this case none of the energy applied to the spine can be absorbed by resilient structures. The most frequent injuring forces are flexion alone and flexion combined with rotation. Injury by extension is much less frequent.

Fracture by flexion. The cause is a fall on to the shoulders or a weight falling on to them and the impact often causes bruises or grazes, which, taken with the history, should arouse suspicion, especially in the unconscious or otherwise uncommunicative patient. A simple wedge fracture, which is quite common in the mid-thoracic region, will cause little swelling because the posterior soft tissues may be stretched but will not be torn; there would, however, be local tenderness. The slight

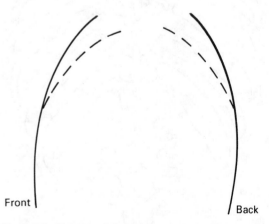

Front   Back

Figure 8.5. Fracture of the sternum by bowing usually means that there is also a fracture of the thoracic part of the spine

accentuation of the normal curvature may escape the untrained eye even in a thin person and in a bulky person any swelling or deformity is even less easy to identify. If there is a large component of longitudinal compression in the injuring force as well as flexion, the upper vertebra may be displaced backwards on the lower and damage the spinal cord. In such cases there may be fractures of the articular facets (Figure 8.6) or the neural arches although in radiographs they are likely to be obscured by the overlying ribs. Burst fractures such as occur in the neck (Figure 2.8) are rare in the thoracic vertebrae.

Fracture by flexion and rotation. This type of injury is caused by much greater forces that are applied on one or other side of the spine. The usual result is fracture-dislocation with damage to the spinal cord and extensive tearing of muscles, ligaments and the thoracic fascia. This causes marked and often extensive swelling with a palpable gap in the line of the spinous processes and their connecting ligaments and in the thoracic fascia (Figure 8.7). There is also tearing of the soft tissues in front of the spine with bleeding into the mediastinum, which may as a result be sufficiently widened to suggest rupture of the aorta. A useful guide, but not an absolute rule, is that if radiographs show that the trachea is not displaced to the right in both the neck and the chest, it is unlikely that the aorta has been ruptured. It

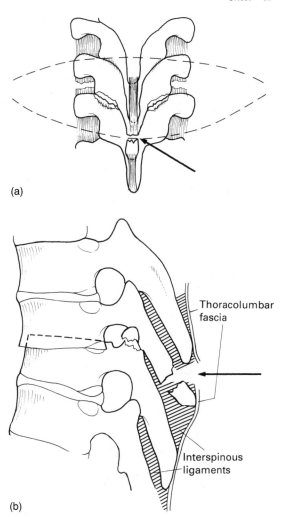

(a)

(b)

Figure 8.7. Fracture-dislocation: a, anteroposterior view; - - - - - represents the edges of the torn thoracic fascia; b, lateral view. The arrows show where a finger easily feels the gap

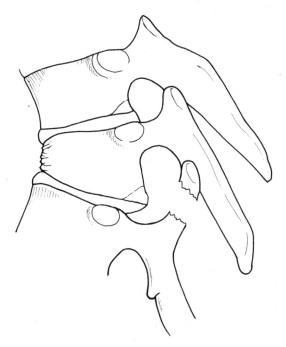

Figure 8.6. Encroachment on the vertebral canal by backward displacement of a vertebra

should be mentioned, however, that a combination of fracture-dislocation and rupture is rare and is likely to be rapidly fatal (page 67).

The radiographic appearance of fracture-dislocation sometimes shows the upper segment to be offset both sideways and backwards on the lower (Figure 8.8) and this may seem difficult to reconcile with injury by flexion and rotation. It must be remembered, however, that radiographs show the position in which the components come to rest and not the position of their greatest displacement. Bearing this in mind, Figure 8.9 provides an explanation. Marked rotation can take the upper vertebra sideways off the lower one and would also set the front edge of the upper vertebra behind that of the lower. The springiness of the undamaged part of the rib cage may then be sufficient to correct some of the rotation but little or none of either the descent or the two offsets.

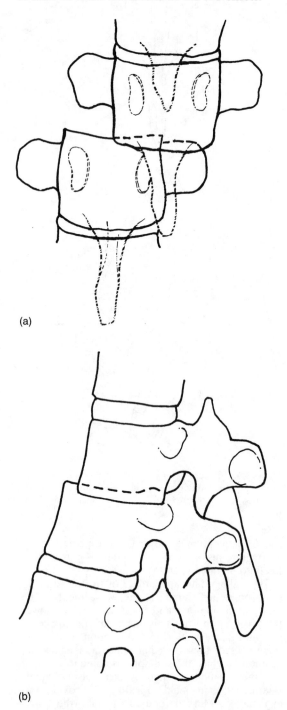

(a)

(b)

Figure 8.8. Posterolateral displacement with fracture-dislocation of thoracic vertebrae: a, anteroposterior view; b, lateral view

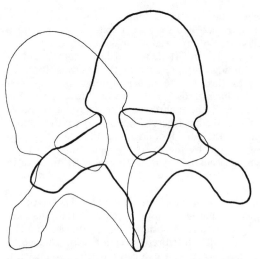

Figure 8.9. Effect of marked rotation on the relative positions of two thoracic vertebrae. Accompanying fractures have not been represented

Fracture by extension is rare. It can result from falling backwards over a ridge or bar or from violent impact as in a road accident, when it may be accompanied by rupture of the descending part of the aorta.

Injuries of soft tissues

Injuries of muscles

These are inevitable with fractures and dislocations but in old persons ribs can be broken so easily that the intercostal muscles suffer little or no damage. As a result, they continue to provide sufficient splintage to hold the broken ends together and so prevent paradoxical movement. Over the course of a week or so, however, the elastic recoil of the lungs and perhaps the weight of the forequarter can cause sufficient subsidence to produce a striking deformity that is remarkable also for the small effect it has on comfort and breathing.

Injuries of viscera

The heart can be injured by impact or crushing. Direct impact can bruise the myocardium and cause a haemopericardium as well as some infarction of the muscle. It can also lead to contusion and thrombosis of a coronary artery, with more severe and extensive ischaemia of the myocardium. Distortion of the heart by crushing can rupture septa, valves or chordae tendineae, with consequent reflux, systolic murmurs and acute heart failure. The precise site and nature of the injuries owe something to the phase of the cardiac cycle, and perhaps of respiration, at the moment of injury and are not solely the result of the injuring force.

The pericardium can be torn by distortion of the chest, either as part of the diaphragm or beside the heart and it has been known for the heart to be forced out through the rent but still acting and capable of recovering after being replaced (King and Sapsford, 1978; Clifford, 1984).

The trachea and bronchi are torn by shearing forces. The flexible chest of a child can be so deeply indented without fracture that the main bronchus can be severed, indeed a lung can be torn off, without any external sign of injury. In adults, fracture of the front part of the fifth rib is sometimes associated with rupture of the right main bronchus and can be a useful warning that this may have occurred.

Ruptures of these large air passages cause surgical emphysema that appears first at the root of the neck, having tracked upwards through the mediastinum.

The aorta. Rupture of the aorta occurs typically between the subclavian artery and the ligamentum arteriosum, where it is the result of violent stretching when inertia or other displacing force shifts the heart and the arch of the aorta suddenly towards the head. It is almost confined to persons in motor vehicles. The rupture varies from a small tear in front to complete transection. If the adventitia remains intact, as it may do, the victim can survive, even without surgical repair but with a false aneurysm. This injury is well known for having little or no sign of external injury in some cases. A rare sign, paraplegia, results from dissection within the wall of the vessel that obstructs the arteries that supply the spinal cord. Sometimes dissection compresses the subclavian artery and makes the blood pressure in the left arm lower than that in the right.

Rupture of the descending part of the aorta occurs much less often than the above. It is associated with extension fracture-dislocation of the spine in pedestrians that have been struck by motor vehicles (Sevitt, 1977). It is also one of the fatal injuries of the victims of aircraft crashes who are thrown forwards over their seat belts.

Rupture of the ascending aorta is rarer still; it occurs above the aorta's valves and is the result of impact directly over it (Sevitt, 1977).

The oesophagus can be torn by severely displaced fractures but the victim would be unlikely to survive the associated injuries.

The lungs. Injuries are usually inflicted by broken ribs but troublesome bleeding is much more likely to come from the chest wall than from the lung. Air escapes through the torn tissues to reach the fascial and subcutaneous planes near the site of injury, from where it may then spread widely and rapidly. Its spread is limited above by the fusion of the two layers of the superficial fascia at the level of the eyebrows and the temporal line and below at the groins but it can spread into the arms and also into the genitals. It is less well known, although it has long been known (Maclin, 1939), that air can spread into the pericardial or the peritoneal cavity, although this is rare. The air passes from the torn alveoli along the blood vessels of the lung to the mediastinum and thence to one or other cavity, even though the peritoneum may appear to be intact. This process is assisted by artificial ventilation with fairly high inflation pressure.

Blast. Injury of the lungs by blast has become a noteworthy condition for clinicians since explosions have become more frequent. The blast wave travels at the speed of sound from its source; if it passes from water into air it causes a low, dome-like raising of the surface of the water and this is accompanied by small jet-like projections and drops thrown from the surface – an occurrence known as spalling (Rawlings, 1978). When a blast wave passes through the chest, the interface between gas and liquid in the alveoli is subjected to this disruptive process, which results in haemorrhagic congestion of the lung and consequent hypoxaemia. The pleural surface of one or both lungs may also be torn, which means that however necessary artificial ventilation may be to correct hypoxaemia, it can cause rapidly enlarging and bilateral pneumothoraces unless the cavities are adequately vented. These changes may occur very quickly or not for 24 h or so; the interval is presumably determined by the force of the explosion and whether or not it occurs within a confined space.

If examined post mortem, the lungs are heavy and wet and may show purplish stripes that appear to correspond with the ribs; in fact they correspond with the intercostal spaces. This is because at the moment of exposure to the blast wave the ribs provide protective support for the lungs but there is sudden congestion of the unsupported parts between the ribs.

The diaphragm. Two forces can tear the diaphragm: one is violent distortion of the chest; the other is a sudden rise in pressure within the abdomen, but it may be impossible to separate the one from the other and the two can occur together.

A heavy blow that breaks an arm when it is beside the chest, and tears both the diaphragm and the spleen, acts by distortion, whereas a crush injury that breaks the pelvis may also distort the chest or raise intra-abdominal pressure or both. The phase of respiration may also play a part in that a tense diaphragm is more likely to split when it is distorted and a slack one to be burst by a sudden rise in pressure. Most ruptures are more or less radial in the muscular part of the diaphragm but occasionally the central tendon is torn. Although it has often been stated that rupture rarely affects the right side of the diaphragm, this may not be so. Ruptures on the right side can be plugged by the liver so that no herniation of gut occurs and the condition goes unrecognized.

Wounds

Wounds may accompany any of the injuries that have already been described but many are the result of stabbing, and penetrate rather than disrupt. It should be remembered that penetrating wounds between the nipples and the navel may enter the chest or the belly or both and that some require immediate operation to deal with bleeding from the heart or a large blood vessel. Stab wounds that pierce the diaphragm may give little sign of their existence and can consequently be overlooked but they are noteworthy because the small hole can be gradually enlarged by the movements of the diaphragm and perhaps by the fluctuating pressure of respiration, with the result that months or years later herniation and strangulation of abdominal organs can occur.

Penetration by high-velocity missiles (travelling at >1100 feet per second; ≈330 m s^{-1}) causes severely disruptive wounds with no characteristic patterns except that the lungs absorb little energy from the missile and consequently suffer less damage than more solid structures. The passage of a high-velocity missile causes the formation of a temporary cavity with a diameter that may be as much as 30 times the calibre of the missile. This is the result of the shock wave that precedes the missile and it causes severe damage in the distorted tissues. The amount of damage done to the tissues through which the missile passes depends on the kinetic energy ($\frac{1}{2}mv^2$) that they absorb. This in turn depends on the density of the tissue and upon the shape and size of the missile: large and irregular ones will slow down much more quickly and give up more energy than small and smooth missiles (Owen-Smith, 1981). The disruptive effect of such missiles has given rise to accusations that explosive bullets have been used.

Once the cavity created by the passage of the missile has collapsed, it may not be evident to the inexperienced eye just how severe and extensive the damage has been and how much tissue needs to be removed by the surgeon.

Low-velocity missiles behave in quite a different way. They do not cause cavitation and consequently they do little damage except to the tissues with which they come into contact. They may not follow a direct path from the point of entry to the place of lodgement or exit because they can be deflected along tissue planes and travel, for example, in the thickness of the chest wall.

Abdomen

Fractures and dislocations

Fractures of the ribs

There is little to add to the account given of these injuries in the chest but it is worth remarking that fractures of the tenth rib may be associated with ruptures of the spleen, liver or kidney. A heavy blow landing behind the liver can not only pulp part of that organ but may tear hepatic veins as the liver is displaced by the impact. In the circumstances, the combination of marked pallor, a distended belly and a limp patient is strongly suggestive of very severe internal bleeding and calls urgently for massive infusion of blood, followed by exploration.

Fractures of the spine

Wedge fractures are common but not usually serious.

The thoracolumbar junction is most often the site of serious injury in this part of the spine. Much of what has already been stated about fractures and dislocations on pages 64–66 applies but some points of difference deserve attention.

Injuries below the first lumbar vertebra. Because the spinal cord ends at the lower border of the first lumbar vertebra, fracture-dislocations lower down can injure only nerve roots, which, unlike the cord, are capable of regeneration.

Fracture-dislocations are usually accompanied by tearing of the posterior soft tissues, with swelling and a palpable gap both in the lumbar fascia and between the spinous processes. There is, however, a pattern of injury in which the back of the neural arch remains in place and separation takes place in the region of the pedicles (Figure 8.10). This means that the interspinous ligaments and the lumbar fascia remain intact. An anteroposterior radiographic view shows what at first sight may appear to be a typical fracture-dislocation, perhaps with a wedge of bone broken from one vertebral body (the so-called slice fracture) but careful examination will identify the fact that although there

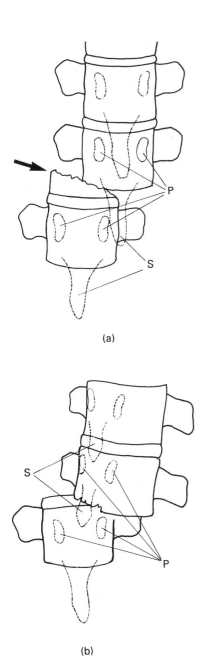

(a)

(b)

Figure 8.10. Contrasting patterns of fracture-dislocation in the lumbar spine. a, The usual pattern of fracture-dislocation by flexion and rotation; the pedicles P and the spinous processes S are offset above the fracture. b, The spinous processes are not offset with the bodies of their vertebrae; the pedicles may or may not be

important difference in a jumble of bony shadows is not recognized, and if the back is not examined carefully with the fingers, a fruitless attempt at posterior stabilization may be undertaken.

Locked facets. Occasionally, flexion with some distraction causes dislocation and locking of the facets but in this part of the spine the shape and arrangement of the articular facets are such that unilateral dislocation cannot occur without fracture (Figure 8.11).

Hyperextension injuries are rare; they occur between the facets and the body of the vertebra and

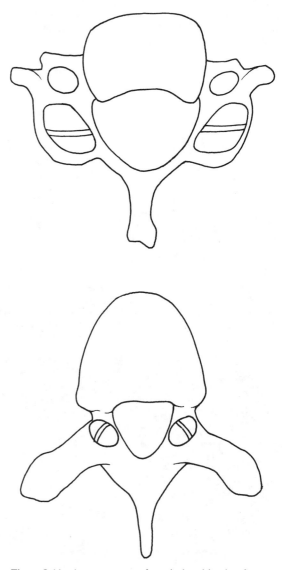

is some irregularity, the general line of the spinous processes is unbroken. Depending on where the fracture occurs, the pedicles may remain with either the spinous processes or the bodies or they may be partly with each (Figure 8.10b). If this

Figure 8.11. Arrangements of cervical and lumbar facets

if there is little displacement they may permit immediate cautious activity by the patient. It should be noted that marks of a blow on the back can occur with both flexion and extension injuries; the differences are shown by Figure 8.12.

Fractures of transverse processes are almost always traction injuries and they can fairly be regarded and treated as torn muscles. The thick padding of muscles behind them makes it unlikely that the force of even a heavy blow would carry through to the transverse processes.

Chance's fracture passes horizontally through a spinous process and is the result of distraction with some flexion such as could result from an impact directed towards the head.

Injuries of the soft tissues

Muscles

These are torn by fractures but a heavy blow on the iliac crest can shear the muscles from it; it may not break the skin, so that unless the area is palpated carefully, swelling may mask the defect in the muscles – another example of a soft-centred bruise.

When the abdominal muscles are contracted they provide excellent protection for the viscera but a heavy blow can drive the relaxed abdominal wall against the spine and crush through some of its muscle (Figure 8.13).

Viscera

Injury by impact. The less mobile parts of the intestine can be injured in the same way and at the

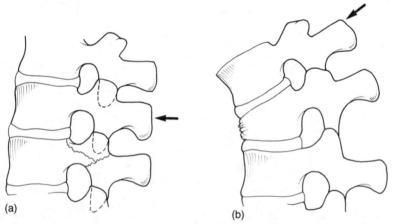

Figure 8.12. Opposite effects of a blow in the back. a, Hyperextension. The anterior longitudinal ligament remains intact and the articular processes of the vertebra above act as fulcra over which the partes interarticulares below can be broken. b, Flexion. The arrows show the sites of both impact and marks of injury

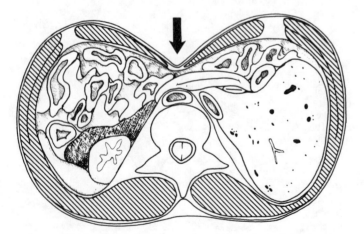

Figure 8.13. Crushing of muscle in the abdominal wall against the spine

same time as muscle (Figure 8.13). In each case, the blow may produce purplish, spotty bruising of the skin and when this mark is present on skin that does not lie directly over bone, however faint and small it may be it warrants exploratory laparotomy unless internal injury can certainly be ruled out. Such injuries range from mere bruising of mesentery, bowel or other organs to severe rupture of the spleen, liver or kidney and transection of the bowel or the pancreas. Careful examination of retroperitoneal haematomata may also show that a suprarenal gland has been torn but rupture of a large retroperitoneal blood vessel by a blow is rare.

The fact that there is a retroperitoneal haematoma calls for care and judgement in deciding whether or not to explore it. Large and spreading ones over the spine are likely to come from large blood vessels and should be explored, with plenty of blood readily available. A rare consequence of a large and tense retroperitoneal haematoma is pressure on the inferior vena cava that is sufficient to cause venous congestion and cyanosis of the lower part of the trunk and the thighs.

Haematomata adjoining bowel should be explored in search of possible tears, but if they are not expanding and if on exploration they appear to have originated from the kidney, further exploration may provoke troublesome bleeding and do more harm than good; the kidney has remarkable powers of recovery and decision can be assisted by angiography, even on the operating table. Angiography can be helpful also when there is a large haematoma in the pelvis, especially when it shows a torn artery that may be treatable by therapeutic embolism.

The influence of hernial orifices. Where the natural support of the abdominal wall is lacking, a sudden rise in pressure within the belly can rupture the gut.

Blast. An explosion under water can burst the intestine of persons in the water (see page 119).

Wounds. Stab wounds can enter the belly from the lower part of the chest, the back, the groins, the buttocks or the perineum, and bullets from more distant places of entry, and they may injure any of the abdominal organs. A blunt object may be driven into the belly and penetrate deeply among the bowels. If it enters the anus it is almost certain to tear the rectum or the pelvic colon but if it pierces the skin, whether in the perineum or elsewhere, it can pass harmlessly among the coils of intestine. There have been numerous examples of impalement and even transfixion by blunt objects in which the only serious damage has been confined to the places of entry and exit.

Stab wounds cause internal injury in only about 50% of cases. The explanation is that even a sharp object can push the slack belly wall inwards before piercing it. This displaces the gut and when the weapon does pierce the belly wall this slides back along the blade, staining it for perhaps several inches, while the displaced viscera move gently and harmlessly into contact with the weapon.

A good deal of attention has been devoted to deciding whether or not to explore stab and similar penetrating wounds. It has been suggested that the decision should be based on whether or not the peritoneum has been breached. This is an unreliable test for two reasons: the first has already been mentioned, namely that only about 50% of wounds that have entered the peritoneal cavity have damaged viscera; the second is that the track of the weapon that has damaged viscera may then be broken up by the differential movement of the layers of the abdominal wall; the victim will be examined while lying on the back but may have been stabbed while crouching. I have known wounds of the skin, muscle layer and peritoneum to be as much as 2 inches ($\approx$15 mm) apart in each layer. Probing and sinography may therefore give a dangerously misleading impression of the severity of the injury.

Uterus. Until pregnancy causes it to protrude above the brim of the pelvis, the uterus is very unlikely to be injured. As it comes to occupy more and more of the abdominal cavity if offers increasing protection to the mother's viscera, while leaving the child she carries more at risk from both closed and penetrating injuries.

References

Clifford, R. P. (1984) Traumatic rupture of the pericardium with dislocation of the heart. *Injury*, **16**, 123

King, J. B. and Sapford, R. N. (1978) Acute rupture of the pericardium with delayed dislocation of the heart. *Injury*, **9**, 303

Maclin, C. C. (1939) Transport of air along sheaths of pulmonic blood vessels from alveoli to mediastinum: clinical implications. *Archives of Internal Medicine*, **64**, 913

Owen-Smith, M. S. (1981) *High Velocity Missile Wounds*, Edward Arnold, London

Rawlings, J. S. P. (1978) Physical and pathophysiological effects of blast. *Injury*, **9**, 313

Sevitt, S. (1977) Traumatic ruptures of the aorta: a clinicopathological study. *Injury*, **8**, 159

9

The pelvis and hip joints

Pelvis

Minor fractures

The word minor refers to the severity of the injury in relation to function, not to the size of the fracture, which may be extensive (Figure 9.1).

Fractures 1, 2 and 3 (Figure 9.1)

These are avulsion fractures of, respectively, the iliac spines and the tuberosity of the ischium and they occur in vigorous, usually male, patients before the epiphyses have fused. Occasionally they have troublesome after-effects because bone forms in the gap and creates a sizeable prominence.

Fracture 4 (Figure 9.1)

Fractures of the blade of the ilium are the result of a heavy blow; they sometimes run horizontally rather than vertically.

Fracture 5 (Figures 9.1 and 9.2)

The cause is a fall on to the hip; sometimes both pubes are affected. It is an injury of old and elderly women and it owes this fact to the shape of the female pelvis (Figure 9.2).

Fracture 6 (Figure 9.1)

Transverse fractures of the sacrum are rare and are probably the result of a heavy blow on the lower part of the bone. In spite of the large size of the sacral foramina the nerves may be injured by fractures running across the foramina.

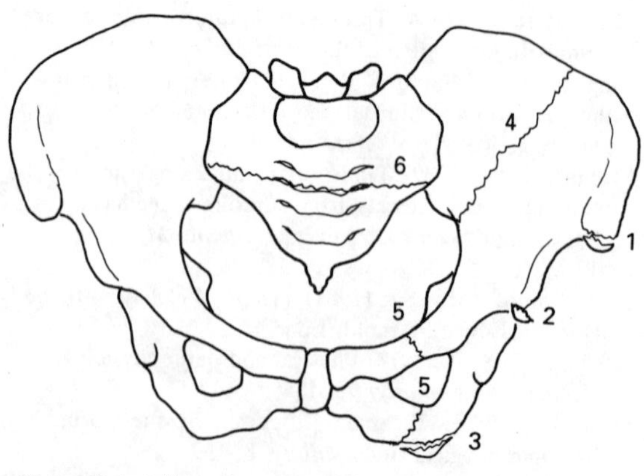

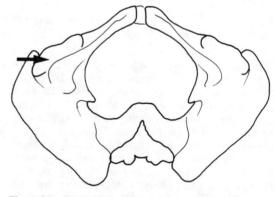

Figure 9.1. Minor fractures of the pelvis. See text for explanation

Figure 9.2. The female pelvis from below. This view makes it easy to understand that a blow directed into the acetabulum can break the narrow rami of the pubis

Fractures of the coccyx

The combination of a blow, tenderness over the coccyx, pain when it is moved by a finger and thumb and sharp forward inclination of the bone is often regarded as grounds for diagnosing fracture of the coccyx. Unequivocal radiological evidence of fracture of the bone is not usual and it may be much less frequent than the diagnosis.

Major fractures

These fall into five groups, which are illustrated by Figure 9.3a–e.

Group A (Figure 9.3a)

These fractures are rare; they occur in younger persons whose bones are strong enough to resist pressure from one or both sides rather than the brief impact of a fall on to the hip. The symphysis gives way and allows the pubes to overlap. This is likely to be accompanied by some damage at the sacroiliac joint on the injured side.

Group B (Figure 9.3b)

Anteroposterior compression can split the pubic symphysis and according to the extent of separation at the symphysis there is more or less damage in the sacroiliac regions, usually fracture of the sacrum or the ilium rather than dislocation of the joint. The opening up of the pelvis resembles that of a book. The extreme example of this pattern of

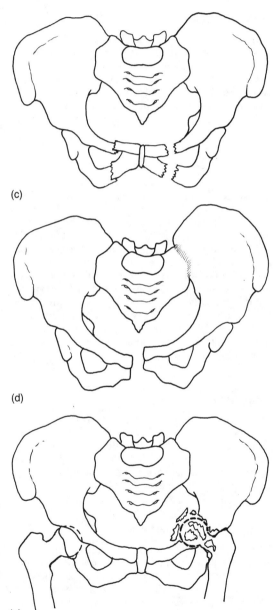

(c)

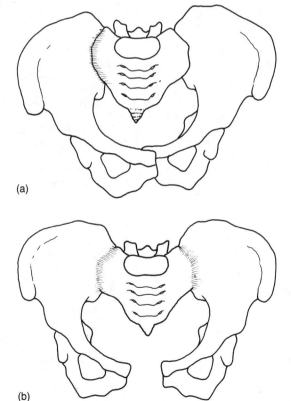

(a)

(b)

(d)

(e)

Figure 9.3. Groups of major fractures of the pelvis. a, Group A: compression with overlap: b, group B: split front; c, group C: displaced pubes; d, group D: upwards dislocation; e, group E: stove-in hip. Shading indicates damage in the sacroiliac region

injury is traumatic amputation of the hindquarter, which, however, is not the result of compression but of violent abduction exerted either through the femur or directly by a blow on the front of the pelvis.

Fractures in groups A and B are not usually accompanied by injuries of the viscera because the bone is peeled away from them.

Group C (Figure 9.3c)

A heavy blow directed backwards in the region of the symphysis can disconnect the pubes from the ischia and the ilia and in so doing it may rupture the bladder or the urethra. A full bladder may burst into the peritoneal cavity as a result of the impact but whether the bladder is full or empty its extraperitoneal part can be punctured by bony spikes.

Group D (Figure 9.3d)

The cause is a more or less vertical upwards force applied to one side of the pelvis, as by a heavy fall on to one buttock, but a heavy blow on the front of one side of the pelvis, as in a road accident, could produce a unilateral variety of a fracture in group B. The circumstances of injury are not usually sufficiently well known to allow the precise manner of injury to be worked out. The viscera often escape damage but it has been known for either large or small bowel to be trapped in a fracture, which may be in the region of the acetabulum, the sacroiliac joint or the blade of the ilium (Lunt, 1970).

Group E (Figure 9.3e)

The appearance in an anteroposterior radiograph is responsible for the widely used term central dislocation of the hip, but the results of more detailed study suggest that stove-in hip is more appropriate and this group is considered separately and in more detail (pages 76–79).

Open fractures of the pelvis

These are usually extremely severe injuries in which the pelvis is more or less shattered, as when it is run over by a heavy vehicle or is trapped in a narrow space between a wall and a moving object. There is extensive flaying of the trunk, buttock and thighs and the wide disruption of the pelvis may cause the rectum and the anus to be torn loose and retract into the cavity. Other viscera are also likely to be seriously damaged.

Hip joint
Fracture-dislocations of the hip
Minor fractures of the acetabulum

Posterior dislocation. Depending on the degree of abduction of the hip, a blow on the knee when the hip is flexed will either displace the head of the femur backwards over the rim or the acetabulum or cause it to break a piece off the rim (Figure 9.4). Young children's hips dislocate more easily than those of adults: a fall on to the knee may be sufficient to put the hip out of joint. Women are more likely to sustain dislocation than fracture-dislocation because their pelves are wider and they usually sit with their knees together, or often with their legs crossed, especially when they are passengers in motor cars.

The blow that dislocates the hip may graze or wound the knee and fracture the patella or the femur, which makes a characteristic pattern of injury.

A commonly recommended method of replacing a dislocated hip is to lie the victim supine on the floor and pull upwards on the thigh with the knee and the hip flexed to right angles. This is not always successful and it ignores the fact that when a hip goes out of joint it is likely to be flexed some way above a right angle, with the thigh even in contact with the trunk. That is because the victim is not sitting upright at the moment of injury; the body is thrown forwards by its inertia whereas the thigh is kept more or less in place by the contact between the knee and the dashboard or a similar structure. The thigh may also be fairly well adducted and medially rotated at the moment of dislocation.

If these possibilities are taken into consideration it may be found that the act of replacement is much less strenuous than had been expected but,

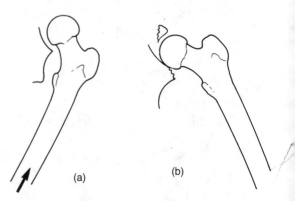

(a) (b)

Figure 9.4. a, With the hip in adduction, dislocation occurs without fracture; b, with the hip in abduction, dislocation is accompanied by fracture

as with the shoulder and the elbow, for example, the position usually has to be altered slightly more than once before exactly the right one is found.

Three other practical matters deserve attention. First, fracture-dislocation may not lock the hip in the familiar position of flexion, adduction and medial rotation and in an unconscious person there may be a good range of passive movement. If there are other fractures in the limb, any shortening at the hip may be blamed on the other fracture(s). A particularly treacherous combination is that of dislocation of the hip with fracture of the shaft of the femur on the same side. To avoid overlooking the dislocation: (a) think of the possibility after any forcible blow on the knee, especially if it does obvious damage at the knee; (b) think of the possibility when there is wide displacement of a fracture of the shaft of the femur. Careful examination of radiographs of the thigh may identify flexion and adduction of the proximal fragment; (c) radiograph the hip joint.

Secondly, manipulation may fail. This may be because it was not properly carried out; it may be because the damage to the acetabulum renders it unstable and in need of surgical reconstruction, or it may be because soft tissues obstruct the return of the head to its socket. Although exploration has sometimes shown this to be the case, one may justifiably wonder whether just the right position of the hip was found by the manipulator rather than that the dislocation was really 'valvular' and uncorrectable without an operation.

Thirdly, manipulation may seem to have succeeded. It may be taken for granted that the hip will be radiographed after manipulation but it needs to be stated that both hips should be, and on the same film. This is because flakes of bone or cartilage or part of the capsule may be trapped in the joint. Although they cast no shadow on the film, they will make the joint slightly less than congruous but unless both hips appear on the same film the slight difference from normal may well go unrecognized.

When the rim of the acetabulum has been broken, it matters less whether or not the fragment resumes its rightful place after manipulation, than whether or not the hip can be easily put out of joint again when it is slightly more adducted than it would be in a standing or a sitting position.

Fracture of the head of the femur sometimes occurs in the course of posterior dislocation of the hip and may therefore be considered here rather than with other fractures of the femur. This type of fracture is rare; usually the fragment is no more than a thick slice from the medial aspect of the head, being sheared off by the edge of the acetabulum. It does not form part of the weight-bearing surface of the head, so that it if does not lie

accurately in place after manipulation it can safely be moved. If it does lie accurately in place this may be because it has been retained by the ligamentum teres and may have a sufficient blood supply for the fracture to unite.

Rarely, and usually in young persons (because it requires great violence), the whole head of the femur, and sometimes the neck as well, is broken off.

Viability of the head of the femur after dislocation of the hip. It has often been stated that there is serious risk of avascular necrosis after dislocation and that osteoarthritis will follow but a careful study of more than 100 hips for at least 3 years after dislocation yielded only two examples of this complication (Proctor, 1973). Although any blood supplied to the head by the ligamentum teres is certainly cut off, the main blood supply of the head of the femur (Figure 9.5) comes from vessels that are derived from the circumflex femoral arteries and these pass through tissues that are displaced rather than torn when the hip is dislocated.

Anterior dislocation of the hip is much rarer than posterior and, when there is a clear account of how it happened, forcible abduction with more or less lateral rotation of the femur is responsible.

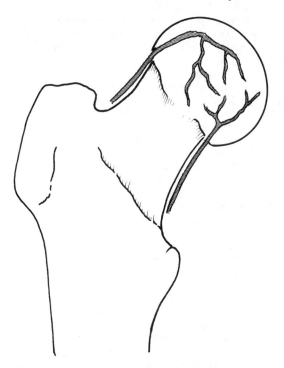

Figure 9.5. The head of the femur is supplied mainly by the lateral and medial epiphyseal arteries, which run along the neck from its base

The head of the femur is usually levered forwards out of its socket without demonstrable fracture of either, but sometimes the front of the rim is broken and this can make it easy for dislocation to recur if the limb rolls outwards when the patient is lying down. Sometimes the limb lies on its outer side, widely abducted and also flexed at the hip and the knee, which may show marks of injury on its inner side. Alternatively, the limbs are more or less together but with the dislocated one lying on its outer side. In this case, the head of the femur may cause a visible prominence in the groin and press on the femoral vein, so causing venous congestion of the limb. If this does occur, it subsides as soon as displacement is corrected and the pressure thereby relieved.

Stove-in hip

A heavy blow on the knee when the hip is flexed and abducted, or a heavy blow on the side of the hip, can drive the head of the femur into its socket hard enough to break it and the surrounding bone severely and extensively. As seen from the front, the appearance suggests that the head of the femur has been displaced inwards into the pelvis (Figure 9.3e) but extensive surgical experience and suitably directed radiographs have brought understanding and order to what was long regarded as an insoluble bony jigsaw puzzle.

The main patterns of fracture are shown on Figures 9.6 and 9.7. In the individual case the pattern depends on the precise magnitude and direction of force and when the latter acts in the line of the femur it depends on the degrees of flexion and abduction of the hip. Pattern A (Figure 9.6a) is the result of a force with a large backward component and is known as a fracture of the posterior column. In patterns B and C (Figures 9.6b, c) the backward component is roughly matched by the inward one and in pattern D (Figure 9.6d) the force is directed entirely inwards.

Patterns A–E in Figures 9.7a–e are the results of forces with a considerable forward component (F); A (Figure 9.7a) and C (Figure 9.7c) are examples of fractures of the anterior column. The lengths of the arrows are meant to indicate approximately the relative magnitudes of the components of the injuring force; other components may be directed in upward or downward directions.

Identifying the particular fracture is an essential preliminary to an attempt at surgical repair and it depends on the interpretation of oblique views at right angles to each other as well as the anteroposterior view. Figure 9.8 shows the key features of these three views of the pelvis.

Although there are strong ligaments between the femur and the pelvis, even powerful traction on the limb does not usually have any useful effect on the displaced pieces of bone. The usual effect on the head of the femur is to pull it away from the fragments medial to it but as soon as the pull ceases the head sinks back to where it was.

Soft tissues

Wounds

Wounds may accompany any of the injuries of the pelvis, the most severe and extensive being those associated with open fractures (see page 74).

Bleeding

The most frequent serious effect of fractures of the pelvis is bleeding, which can amount to several times the normal blood volume of the injured person. Even mild fractures of the pubes in old persons can give rise to signs of exsanguination. Some bleeding is from the bone itself, a good deal comes from the torn connective tissues and any injured organs but the most severe bleeding comes from veins and arteries torn by the fractures. These are usually vessels such as the superior gluteal, obturator and internal pudendal arteries, which run close to bone (Figure 9.9). The recommendation that their parent vessel, the internal iliac artery, be ligated as a means of stopping severe bleeding is not reliable. That is because blood vessels that lie within the pelvis but are not pelvic vessels in the ordinary sense, e.g. those in the mesentery, can be torn by spikes of bone; furthermore, occasionally abdominal injuries that are not the result of fracture of the pelvis coexist and cause serious bleeding. For this reason, whenever possible, angiography should be used before undertaking exploration; it may be possible to stop the bleeding by therapeutic embolism and even to avoid opening the belly.

Bleeding caused by fractures of the pelvis can fill the cavity of the pelvis and extend upwards as far as the umbilicus in front and the kidneys behind, but it quite often remains extraperitoneal. This means that if injury of abdominal organs is suspected, peritoneal lavage can still be of use: a positive result settles nothing, but a negative one is reassuring.

Viscera

There is nothing to add to previous remarks about ruptures of the bladder, urethra and, much more rarely, the rectum, colon and small bowel. Occasionally the diaphragm is ruptured either by distortion of the trunk as a whole or by a sudden rise in pressure within the belly.

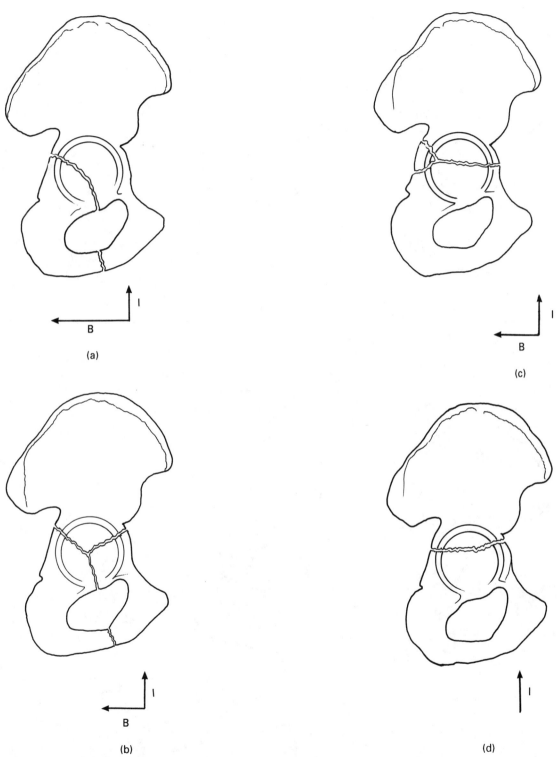

Figure 9.6. Patterns of posterior injuries in which the inward component of the injuring force is least in (a) and greatest in (d). The lengths of the arrows represent inward (I) and backward (B) components of the force; they indicate approximate magnitudes and are not to scale

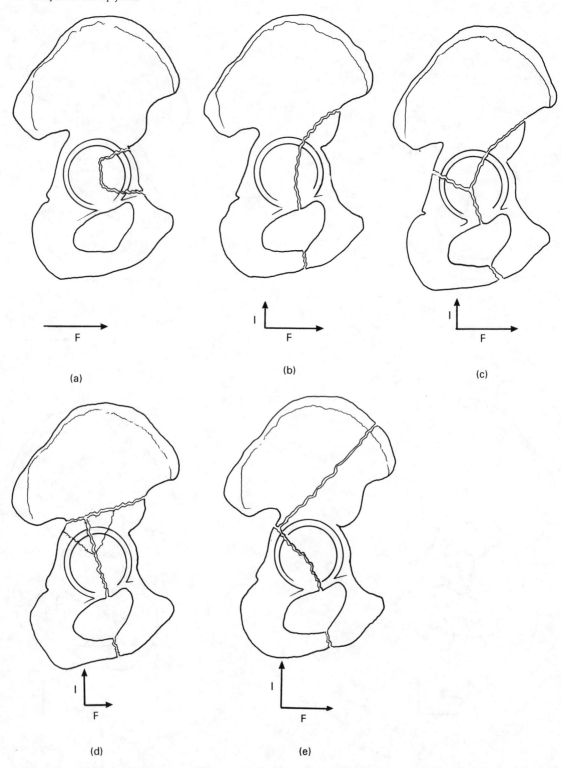

Figure 9.7. Patterns of injury in which there is a strong forward (F) component of the injuring force. I, inward component

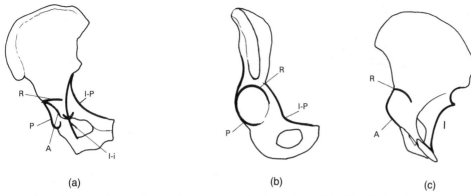

Figure 9.8. Outlines of the radiographic appearances in three views of the hip; the key features are emphasized. a, Anteroposterior view; b, patient recumbent and rolled 45 degrees away from the injured side; c, patient recumbent and rolled 45 degrees towards the injured side. A, Anterior edge of acetabulum; I, posterior edge of innominate bone; I-i, ilioischial line; I-P, iliopectineal line; P, posterior edge of acetabulum; R, roof of acetabulum

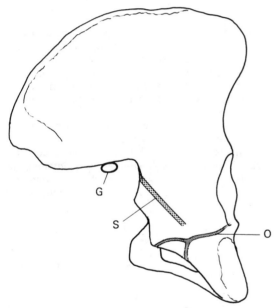

Figure 9.9. Back view of right hip bone: G, superior gluteal artery; O, obturator artery; S, sciatic nerve

Pregnancy

Serious injury during pregnancy is rare but it can result in rupture of the uterus. Although the child may still be alive when the victim reaches hospital, its own injuries are likely to make even urgent laparotomy fruitless. Quite a different sort of injury can also kill an unborn child: when the head is engaged in the pelvis the skull can be broken by even a mild-looking adjoining fracture of the iliopubic region.

Nerves

Although they are large and run close to bone in places, the main nerves in the pelvis are not often injured by fractures. The most frequent injury is of the sciatic nerve by fracture of the back of the acetabulum (Figure 9.9). The nerve is most likely to be frayed or split by a sharp edge of bone but I have known it to be trapped in a fracture of the ischium. I have also known the sciatic nerve to be trapped in a great sciatic notch that had been greatly narrowed by a fracture in group D (Figure 9.3).

More frequent, and in many ways of much greater importance, is the damage to the autonomic nerves that can result in impotence, which may be permanent.

References

Lunt, H. R. W. (1970) Entrapment of bowel within fractures of the pelvis. *Injury*, **2**, 121

Proctor, H. (1973) Dislocations of the hip joint (excluding 'central dislocations') and their complications. *Injury*, **5**, 1

10

The hip and thigh

Fractures of the upper end of the femur

Definitions and classifications

Although a good deal of attention has been paid to these subjects they are important only as they help one to understand how best to treat the individual fracture in the individual patient.

Neck of the femur

Three levels of fracture are described, namely, subcapital, midcervical and basal. Fractures of the middle of the neck are extremely rare if one takes care to obtain good radiographs and remembers that altering the line of sight in relation to the neck of the femur can appear to alter the position of the fracture (Figure 10.1), and also that if the head of the femur is flexed in the acetabulum the projection (P) that is often seen on the lower part of the broken surface of the head can be misinterpreted (Figure 10.2). In the same way, the apparent inclination of the fracture to the long axis of the neck varies with the line of sight and invalidates classification into abduction and adduction fractures.

The most useful guide to the prospects of success after keeping the head and fixing it with a view to union of the fracture is provided by Garden's classification (Garden, 1961) (Figure 10.3). The practical value of this classification lies in the fact that stages 1 and 2 offer the best and stage 4 the poorest prospect of stable fixation and union of the fracture, with stage 3 fractures in an intermediate position. Although, at first sight, fractures in stage 3 are more displaced than those in stage 4 and might therefore be expected to fare

worse, the reason why the trabecular pattern has been altered in stage 3 is that the fragments are still connected by soft tissue. As the limb rolls outwards and the neck rotates forwards this connection causes it to pull on and rotate the head. The presence of this connection has the advantage that it enables the two fragments to be locked together when the hinge that it provides is made taut (Figure 10.4). In the absence of the hinge, movements of the distal fragment offer no mechanical assistance in restoring or maintaining a good position of the fracture and the head remains in its natural resting position in the acetabulum.

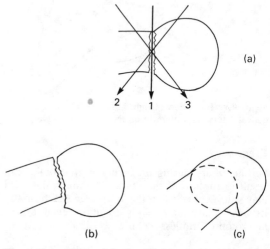

Figure 10.1. Effect of the line of sight on the apparent position of a fracture of the neck of the femur. a, View from above. Line of sight 1 is in the plane of the fracture and provides appearance (b) in the anteroposterior view, whereas the oblique lines of sight 2 and 3 will provide appearance (c)

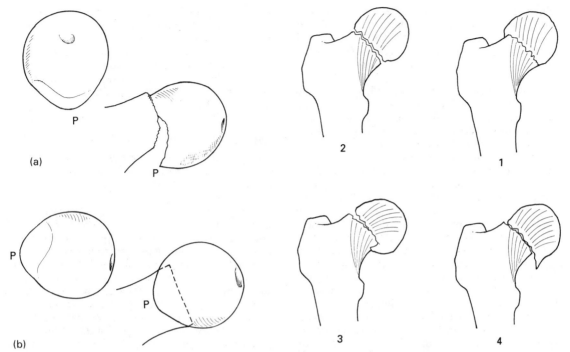

Figure 10.2. The effect of flexion of the head on the femur of the apparent position of a fracture of the neck, which has already allowed the neck to move proximally in relation to the head: the natural (a) and the flexed (b) positions of the head as seen from the side and from the front

Figure 10.3. Garden's classification of subcapital fractures of the femur: stage 1 shows slight abduction at the fracture and the trabecular pattern is altered accordingly; stage 2 shows little more than a crack; in stage 3 the fragments have separated and the trabecular pattern in the head no longer matches that in the neck; in stage 4 the trabecular pattern in the head is the same as that in the neck but it has been shifted downwards with the head

In fact, operations to remove the head of the femur have shown that the radiological difference between fractures of stages 3 and 4 does not always depend on the presence of a hinge.

It should be added that union of the fracture in a good position does not rule out the possibility of avascular necrosis of the head. Any subcapital fracture may tear the blood vessels that enter the holes where the head and the neck join. Even though the head be rendered completely avascular in this way, if it remains in firm contact with the neck this can provide the cells that can join live to dead bone. The later subsidence of the weight-bearing part of the head is not avascular necrosis but a sequel to it and a consequence of the process of revival of the head, whether from the neck, the ligamentum teres or both. Garden (1971) has shown the relevance, to the prospects of achieving

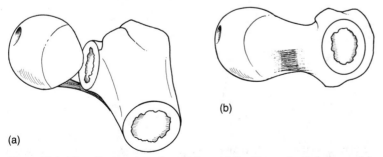

Figure 10.4. The effect, as seen from below, of the hinge of soft tissue on (a) the displacement of a subcapital fracture and (b) its stability after manipulation

bony union of the fracture and retaining a head of normal shape, of the alignment of the head and the neck of the femur; nevertheless, there is still the difficulty that can arise as a result of comminution of the back of the neck of the femur.

How the fracture occurs.   It is well known that the hip is broken by a fall but it is perhaps less well known that the fall is often on to the hip. Evans (1957) showed that both static and dynamic loads applied to either the head or the greater trochanter could break the neck of the femur and there is supporting evidence in the fact that there is sometimes a bruise over the greater trochanter; indeed, this can be a useful warning that posterior comminution of the neck has occurred. Unless a blow on the side of the hip is directed precisely along the neutral axis of the neck of the femur, it will exert a mechanical couple and cause the head to rotate in the acetabulum. If the femur rotates medially the movement will be stopped by the tension of the soft tissues and fracture is unlikely, but if the rotation is lateral the impact of the back edge of the acetabulum can break the neck and it may indent a plate of bone or cause comminution (Figure 10.5). The fact that the head is naturally offset slightly backwards on the neck may play a part in determining the pattern of the fracture because it provides a slightly curved structure that, when loaded from end to end, tends to become more curved and may fail in the process.

The foregoing is not to suggest that all fractures of the neck of the femur are caused by a blow on the side of the hip; a heavy stumble might overload the neck from above, but it could also cause the femur to rotate as described above. There is another way in which the neck can break and that is slowly. This happens when, usually in old persons, the bone becomes just too weak to withstand the loads imposed by standing and walking. There may be a history of a fall but that may be the result and not the cause of the fracture. In such cases, enquiry is likely to disclose that there had

been some discomfort and perhaps stiffness for some time before the fall. This fracture differs from the majority in that, whereas with an acute fracture the neck moves upwards and forwards in relation to the head, with a slow fracture the neck moves only upwards and so leaves the head disposed almost symmetrically on the neck when seen in the lateral view.

The trochanteric region of the femur

Fractures of the greater and lesser trochanters.   As isolated injuries these are rare and are caused by avulsion.

Major fractures of the trochanteric region.   Although these have been divided into intertrochanteric and pertrochanteric types (Figure 10.6), when they are comminuted the distinction is lost. It is therefore reasonable to call them all trochanteric fractures. The patterns of these fractures are shown by Figure 10.7. They can be caused by a blow on the side of the hip. It may be interesting to speculate on why such a blow may break the neck or the trochanteric region of the femur or the pelvis but it is quite likely that one would have to seek an explanation from the precise amount, direction and speed of application of the force as well as from the distribution of strength in the bones concerned.

Fracture (a)   (Figure 10.7a) may be at the base of the neck or a little further laterally and truly pertrochanteric.

Fracture (b)   (Figure 10.7b(i–iii)) is much the

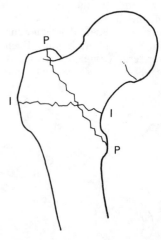

Figure 10.6. Intertrochanteric fractures (I) pass between the greater and the lesser trochanters; pertrochanteric fractures (P) pass through them

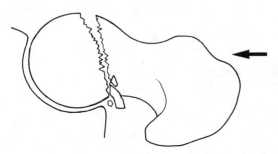

Figure 10.5. A blow on the side of the hip may cause the femur to rotate laterally and the neck to be broken with posterior comminution. Seen from below

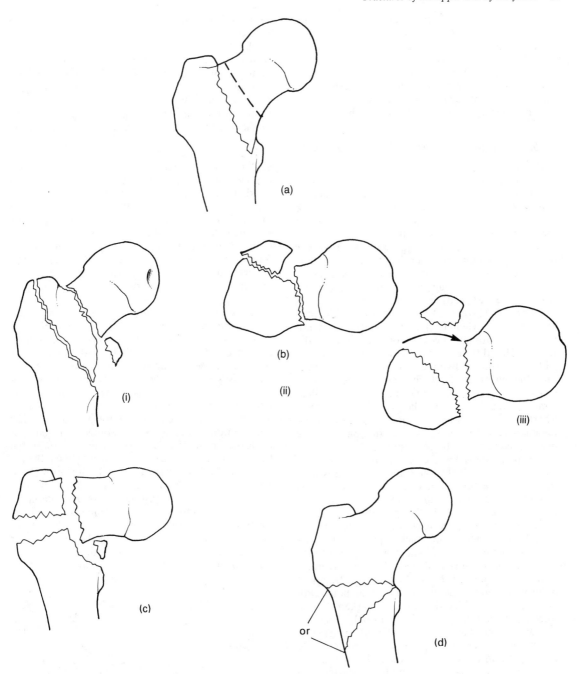

Figure 10.7. Patterns of trochanteric fractures of the femur. Views (a), (c) and (d) are from the front, (b)i is from the back and (b)ii and (b)iii are from above

same as fracture (a) except that the back of the greater trochanter has also been broken, suggesting that it has been split off in the course of

forcible and excessive lateral rotation. Quite often the posterior component of the fracture separates the lesser trochanter as well.

Fracture (c) (Figure 10.7c) combines inter- and pertrochanteric fractures and may be more comminuted than is shown in the diagram.

Fracture (d) (Figure 10.7d) is intertrochanteric and its direction ranges from roughly horizontal to fairly steeply oblique. This pattern may be the result of vertical rather than lateral loading.

Stability and instability of trochanteric fractures

If the concept of stability is based on the ease with which a fracture remains in place, it needs to be acknowledged that there is a range, at one end of which is stability in a good position and at the other is stability in a poor position. An example of the former is a dry stone wall and of the latter a random pile of stones on the ground. Another way of grading stability is according to whether it is associated with acceptable or unacceptable deformity. There is no argument that fractures (c) and (d) (Figure 10.7c, d) are completely unstable. Fracture (a) (Figure 10.7a) is usually stable in a good position when it is pertrochanteric but not when it is through the base of the neck of the femur. The difference arises from the fact that with a simple, i.e. two-piece, pertrochanteric fracture the intact lesser trochanter provides a firm supporting bracket for that part of the calcar femorale that goes with the proximal fragment. There is also a stout posterior hinge of musculotendinous tissue. Fractures at the base of the neck have neither of these supports.

Except perhaps for the lesser trochanter, fracture (b) (Figure 10.7b(i–iii)) can often be restored to a good position by a combination of traction and medial rotation of the limb and may look as though it will be stable in that position. This is not always so and the fracture may subside into varus. This happens when the bracket provided by the lesser trochanter has been lost and the posterior hinge has been torn. With regard to this fracture, it may be mentioned that if the posterior fragment is displaced and loose, firm contact of bone with bone can be achieved only by marked lateral rotation of the femur (Figure 10.7b(iii)). Although it may be possible to reassemble the fragments accurately by using a posterior approach, the prone position is not always practicable for an old person and even the most accurate reconstruction of the fracture will not necessarily make it stable.

The ability to correlate two-plane radiographs with three-plane reality takes time to acquire; it requires a readiness to explore the more complex fractures with both the eyes and the fingers and, most informatively, by dissection post mortem whenever the opportunity arises.

These matters are of obvious practical importance. Attempts to hold unstable fractures in acceptable positions have been based on three methods of treatment.

The first method is to use implants that will withstand the forces acting on this part of the bone. In practice, such implants may be stronger than the bone, with the result that the part in the neck will cut out upwards or the screws in the shaft will pull out. If the bone is stronger than the metal, the implant may bend or even break in the neck of the femur or where it joins the plate.

The second method is to alter the arrangement of the fragments so as to enhance stability to a degree that will protect the implant from being overloaded. In general, these methods depend on increasing valgus between the neck and the shaft of the femur, so that natural forces press the fragments together rather than bending one on the other (Figure 10.8), or on using the shaft of the femur to support the proximal fragment. The lower corner of the neck fragment may be placed within the marrow cavity of the shaft (Figure 10.9).

The third method is to acknowledge that stability depends upon reliable support by one piece of bone for one or more others. Left to the natural influences of muscular activity and gravity, any fracture will settle into a position from which it is least easily disturbed and consequently in which it can be held with the least difficulty. This can be likened to the position of a sleeping dog in that it may not be achieved all at once and once it has been adopted there can be serious disadvantages in disturbing it. If efforts to correct deformity fail because bone or metal fails, what may have been a long and difficult operation will not only have failed but may bring the disaster of deep infection in its train. One may justifiably wonder whether it was worth disturbing the sleeping dog. Fixing fractures of this kind in deformity has the advantages that the operation is unlikely to be either long or complicated, that the patient is likely to walk sooner than when more optimistic methods

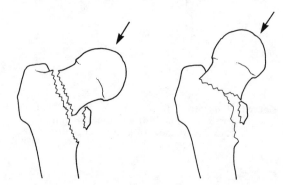

Figure 10.8. Effect of increasing valgus between the neck and the shaft of the femur. The arrows represent the line of weight-bearing

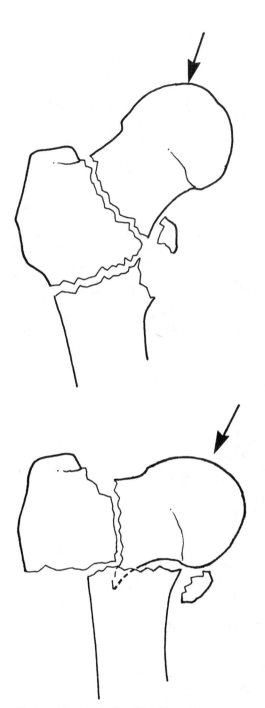

Figure 10.9. Adaptation of McMurray's osteotomy to provide support for the proximal fragment of a comminuted trochanteric fracture

have been used, and that shortening and lateral rotation of the limb are not usually a cause of serious inconvenience, especially when set beside hazards entailed by attempts to achieve something

like anatomical perfection (Verghese and Jaffray, 1987).

Fractures of the trochanteric region of the femur are outstanding examples of the need to understand the pattern of a fracture and, indeed, what may be regarded as the behaviour of a fracture, in order to choose the method of treatment that is likely to be most beneficial to someone who is usually old and often frail as well.

Fractures of the shaft of the femur

The shaft of the femur is here presumed to extend from the lesser trochanter to just above the condyles.

Subtrochanteric fractures

These fractures have powerful abductor muscles above them and powerful adductor muscles below them, and it is possible that the rapid and forceful application of their opposing effects can augment bending forces acting along the length of the femur. Whether they are applied directly or indirectly, transverse, adducting and twisting forces may also be responsible. These fractures are sometimes widely displaced and, whether comminuted or not, they are unstable. There is also the fact that, because the psoas major and iliacus muscles are attached to the lesser trochanter and the adjoining part of the shaft of the femur, the proximal fragment is sharply flexed, as well as being abducted and laterally rotated by the muscles attached to and near the greater trochanter. For these reasons, the secure and accurate apposition of the upper and lower fragments requires surgical fixation.

Another sort of subtrochanteric fracture occurs when the femur is affected by Paget's disease. Whether the disease is of the dense or the more vascular variety, the slight natural curvature of the weakened bone increases and at the same time its flexibility is overtaxed. This latter shows itself as one or more tension cracks in the convex side of the cortex. The increased bowing of the bone may become obvious externally but there may be no discomfort until the partial fracture becomes complete, which can occur without evident cause. Unlike other fractures caused by bending forces, this sort passes straight across the bone, which is partly because the increased curvature of the bone reduces the proportion of its cross-sectional area that is in compression and partly because of increased brittleness. The reason why these fractures occur makes them difficult to treat and this difficulty is increased by the poor capacity that the bone has for healing, especially in the dense variety of the disease.

Other fractures of the shaft of the femur

These are among the most frequent of the serious fractures of the long bones in adults. In children the fractures are usually spiral and heal rapidly and any malunion is largely, if not completely, corrected by remodelling during growth. Very rarely, fractures at the junction of the middle and lowest thirds of the femur damage the femoral artery where it lies close to the bone as it passes through the opening in the adductor magnus to become the popliteal artery.

Being a very strong bone, the normal femur requires great force to break it and for young motor cyclists the necessary force is all too readily available: it may be applied to the right lower limb by an on-coming vehicle or to the left by the motor cycle itself or by an object with which the rider collides. In such cases the fragments are likely to be widely separated; even so, the bone often separates the muscles rather than tearing through them and it is remarkable how frequently the main nerves and blood vessels escape injury (Figure 10.10).

In the worst cases the bone is driven out through the skin and may be stripped bare of all muscular attachment for 6 inches (≈ 152 mm) or more. Part of the shaft may even be snapped off and lost. For those that are familiar only with the well-splinted limbs of patients brought to hospital by ambulance, it is a salutary experience to hear such a statement as 'When I collected my thoughts I noticed that my foot was beside my head. That did not seem right, so I picked it up and put it beside the other one.' Such is the degree of deformity that can occur.

In less severe cases the bone does not pierce the skin but it may come close enough to it to cause a visible bruise; if the bruise is felt, it is found to have a soft centre in which the bone may be easily felt. This has an important practical application if the fracture is to be operated on, because the easiest and safest way to the fracture is not by one of the conventional surgical approaches but through the soft-centred bruise, which is an internal wound of the thigh. Even though this may mean opening the medial side of the thigh, if the

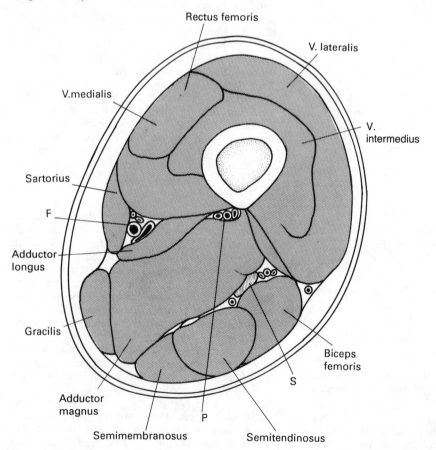

Figure 10.10. Cross-sectional diagram near the middle of the thigh. F, Femoral vessels and branch of nerve; P, profunda femoris vessels; S, sciatic nerve

femoral artery has escaped injury by blindly driven bone it is in no danger from a competent surgeon.

A particularly dangerous set of circumstances is a fracture that causes a good deal of bleeding but is not accompanied by tearing of deep fascia. In such a case the rise in pressure within an inextensible compartment can lead to Volkmann's ischaemia, and the likelihood that it will occur is greater if blood lost from this or other injuries is not adequately replaced. The risk is then of a condition resembling the crush syndrome with renal failure. The condition is very rare but it may face the surgeon with the need to amputate the limb without delay in order to save the patient's life.

For these reasons it will be clear that the damage done to the soft tissues is usually much more important to the surgeon than whether the fracture is transverse, spiral or comminuted or whether it was caused by impact on the thigh or the knee, but it needs to be remembered that several injuries may coexist (Figure 10.11).

Because of the damage to the soft tissues there is usually little difficulty in pulling an adult's femur out to length if it is not to be operated on. Up to 30 lb ($\approx$ 13.5 kg) may be required to achieve the desired length, but 10–15 lb ($\approx$ 4.5–6.75 kg) may then maintain it. This is true even of transverse fractures but it may not be possible to achieve or maintain end-to-end contact by even the most careful application of external splintage. Traction alone is likely to fail when there are fractures at two or more levels because, unless soft tissues connect the fragments, pulling on the distal one will have little or no effect on the proximal and intermediate fragment(s). The tension in the muscles may align the fragment(s) to some extent but there may be large gaps between them (Figure 10.12).

Supracondylar fractures of the femur

In younger persons, whose bones are strong, these fractures are either more or less transverse or they are spiral; they usually result from heavy falls at

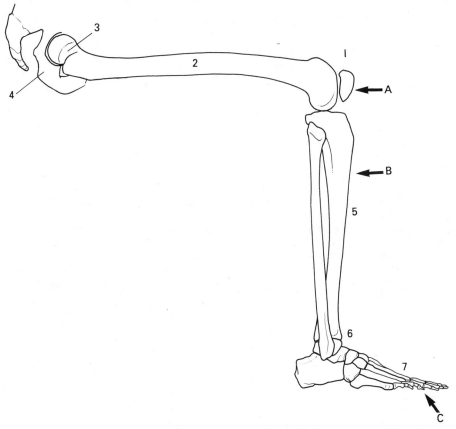

Figure 10.11. Important patterns of injury in the lower limb. The forces represented by the arrows A and B may injure (1) the patella, the lower end of the femur or the knee joint; (2) the shaft of the femur; (3) the neck of the femur; (4) the hip joint, together with (2) (see page 75); (5) the tibia; The impact of the floor, arrow C, may injure (6) the ankle; (7) the foot, or both

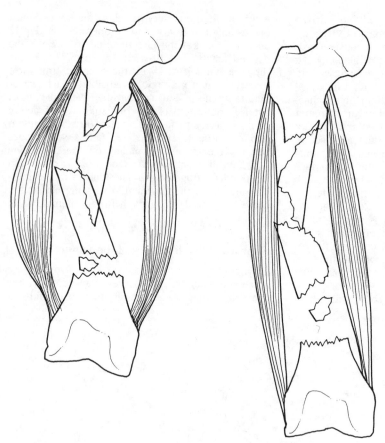

Figure 10.12. Traction on a comminuted fracture may have little effect on the alignment of the fragments

home, during sports or in road accidents. The attachment of the gastrocnemius to the condyles of the femur has been blamed for pulling the distal fragment into flexion at the knee, even when the bone has been pulled out to length (Figure 10.13). This may be so, but for this to happen any hinge has to be at the front. In some cases, however, the fracture has obviously been caused by a flexion rather than an extension force, so that any hinge is

at the back and the front edge of the proximal fragment can do quite serious damage to the extensor apparatus just above the patella. In either case, if surgical fixation is not to be undertaken, it is usually possible to achieve a satisfactory position by means of traction and suitably placed support for the fragments (Figure 10.14).

In old persons, with weaker bones, the relatively strong shaft of the femur sometimes drops be-

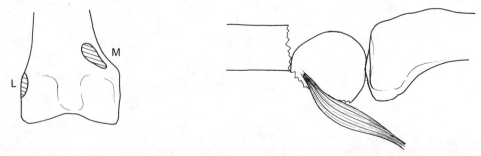

Figure 10.13. Attachments of the gastrocnemius to the femur and their possible effect on it: L, lateral head; M, medial head

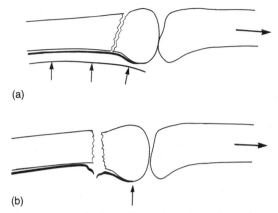

(a)

(b)

Figure 10.14. Beneficial effects of traction and support on (a) flexion and (b) extension types of supracondylar fracture of the femur

tween the condyles and results in what may aptly be likened to a pestle and mortar.

Injuries of soft tissues

All that needs to be added to what has already been written in this chapter relates to rupture of muscles. Almost any muscle in the thigh can be torn by a violent pull and the effects are usually troublesome rather than serious. An exception is the quadriceps muscle, which is vulnerable in the elderly and those whose connective tissues have been weakened, as by rheumatoid disease. The usual cause is missing one's footing. The whole muscle may be torn from the patella but sometimes only the rectus femoris is avulsed. The lesser injury may go unrecognized because the victim can still hobble about and may be able to hold the knee straight against gravity. Although the gap can be felt, it is usually occupied by blood and the proximal bulge made when the avulsed muscle contracts may escape notice. If a flake of bone is pulled from the patella this will facilitate diagnosis.

References

Evans, F. G. (1957) *Stress and Strain in Bones, their Relation to Fractures and Osteogenesis.* Thomas, Springfield

Garden R. S. (1961) Low angle fixation in fractures of the femoral neck. *Journal of Bone and Joint Surgery*, **43B**, 647

Garden R. S. (1971) Malreduction and avascular necrosis in subcapital fractures of the femur. *Journal of Bone and Joint Surgery*, **53B**, 183

Verghese G. B. K. and Jaffray, D. (1987) Should comminuted trochanteric fractures of the hip in the elderly be reduced before fixation? *Injury*, **18**, 270

11

The knee

Fractures

Femur

Fractures of the femur where it is part of the knee joint necessarily affect the condyles (Figure 11.1).

Fracture 1: intercondylar

This is either T- or Y-shaped, according to the direction of the upper component. Occasionally only one condyle is broken off. The cause is impact, either on the patella when the knee is bent (Figure 10.11) or by the tibia when it is more or less straight. In the latter event, particularly, there is often a component of adduction or, more usually, abduction, which causes an obviously asymmetrical lesion. Usually the ligaments remain sufficiently intact to allow simple traction on the tibia to bring the fragments together in a position that may be acceptable.

Fracture 2: osteochondral fracture

This lesion often goes unrecognized until a good deal of bone has been absorbed so as to leave the well-known dense and slightly irregular lenticular fragment that appears to be lying in a well-defined concavity in the medial condyle of the femur – an appearance that gave rise to the belief that it was a degenerative lesion, osteochondritis dissecans. When the knee is open it can be shown that flexion combined with lateral rotation and a small amount of lateral shift (translation) of the tibia brings the site of the lesion into contact with the intercondylar eminence of the tibia. When this apposition occurs with the weight passing through the knee, the resulting impact splits off a small part of the convex bony surface. Even if the cartilage over it remains intact, as bony absorption occurs the repeated slight 'give' of the fragment can cause the cartilage to crack and eventually to give way completely and to become part of a loose body.

Fractures 3 and 4

These are flakes of bone pulled off by the deep parts of the collateral ligaments, which have quite small areas of attachment to the femur.

Fracture 5

The well-known bony strip above the medial condyle of the femur, and known as Pelligrini–Stieda's disease, is not a disease nor, indeed, is it a fracture: it is ossification where the superficial and much longer part of the medial ligament has been pulled off the bone (Figure 11.2). Repeated radiography shows the first faint and ill-defined shadow a fortnight or so after the injury, and during the next few months this becomes larger, denser and better defined.

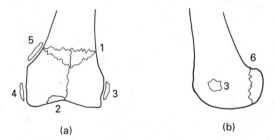

Figure 11.1. Fractures of the condyles of the femur: a, front view; b, side view. For description see text

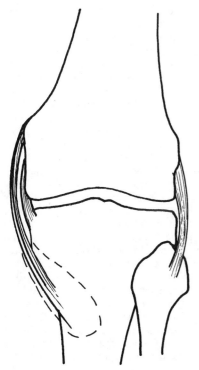

Figure 11.2. Collateral ligaments of the knee joint. The dotted line represents the pes anserinus

Fracture 6

This is a rare injury that resembles the shearing fracture of the capitulum of the humerus (Figure 4.4). The fragment has no soft tissue attached to it and is presumably separated by impact. I have seen three cases. In one of them there was a clear history of sudden severe pain in the knee in the course of a karate kick; the foot was off the ground and had not made contact with its target, which suggests that defective coordination of the muscles acting on the knee allowed the tibia to undergo such forcible translation on the femur as to break off the back of the lateral condyle. In the other two cases the account of the accident was much less informative. What part of the tibia applies the breaking force is a matter for speculation, but when the ligaments have not obviously been torn it seems more likely to be the intercondylar eminence than the edge of the tibia.

Patella

The fractures of the patella are illustrated by Figure 11.3a–c.

Fractures 1 and 2

Most of these are caused by traction, to which may be added the effect of pressure against the femur when the knee is more or less bent. A few result from a blow, in which case there is little or no tearing of the retinacula and consequently little or no separation of the fragments. As the illustration shows, they may affect the articular or the non-articular part of the bone and a few are no more than flakes pulled off in the course of avulsion of the quadriceps. This usually occurs in persons past middle age. The extent of separation of the fragments determines the amount of damage done to the retinacula of the patella.

Fracture 3

This is an avulsion fracture that occurs as the result of displacement of the patella. It is much more likely to be seen from above (Figure 11.3c) than from in front, and when there has been no more than subluxation of the patella it is useful evidence of that displacement. Further evidence is that the medial edge of the bone is tender and pushing the patella laterally makes the patient apprehensive.

Fracture 4

The degrees of both comminution and separation of a stellate fracture depend on the force of a blow on the front of the bone but the exterior apparatus as a whole remains functionally intact.

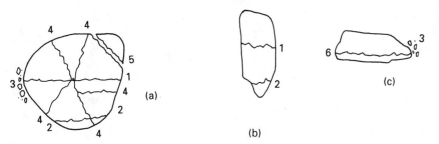

Figure 11.3. Fractures of the patella (a) from behind, (b) from the side, (c) from above. For description see text

Fracture 5

This is usually not a fracture but the gap between the patella proper and a superolateral ossicle, which may be present in both knees. However, a blow may cause tenderness, swelling and an effusion into the knee if it displaces the ossicle.

Fracture 6

A variably sized flake of the articular surface can be sheared off if the patella is displaced sideways while being pressed firmly against the femur.

Tibia

Most of the fractures of the head of the tibia result from either a fall or lateral impact (Figure 11.4).

Fracture 1

This is the most familiar pattern and is caused either by a blow on the outer side of the knee, by

a motor car, for example, or by a fall on to the foot with the knee no more than slightly bent. It usually occurs in persons past middle age. In each case there is a combination of valgus with vertical loading, as a result of which the edge of the lateral condyle of the femur acts as a blunt chisel and splits off the lateral part of the head of the tibia (Figure 11.5a). The degree of damage ranges from little more than a crack to extensive comminution with fragments driven well down into the head of the tibia. The lateral view may show that the depression is posterior rather than anterior or central (Figure 11.4b) and this is because the tibia has been displaced forwards by rotation or by translation. An anteroposterior radiograph may show an appearance such as Figure 11.5b and although I have known a patient to take weight on such a tibia, vertical loading usually causes genu valgum, as in Figure 11.5a. This is of practical importance because it has been stated that obvious valgus instability is an indication for surgical fixation. If, however, such an injury is treated by traction, the fact that the ligaments have remained in continuity, as they usually have, can allow the lateral part of the head of the tibia to be pulled into place and so to support the lateral condyle of the femur once the fracture has united.

Fracture 2

The medial counterpart of fracture 1 does not often occur and when there is direct vertical loading without genu valgum or varum both sides of the head of the tibia can be driven downwards as an inverted T- or Y-fracture.

Fractures of the head of the tibia may be accompanied by crushing or tearing of the meniscus, which may also be buried in the cancellous bone, but they may do little more than tear its peripheral attachment, in which case the meniscus may be retained and repaired.

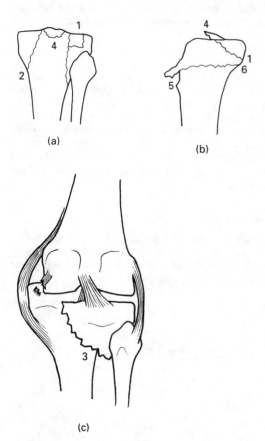

Figure 11.4. Fractures of the upper end of the tibia. For description see text

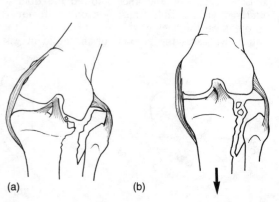

Figure 11.5. Beneficial effects of an intact collateral ligament

Fracture 3

Figure 11.4c shows an unusual variety of fracture 1 in which a large block of the head of the tibia has been displaced in company with the femur. There may be little or no damage to the medial ligament and it may be sufficient to fix the fragment in place for the stability of the joint to be restored.

Fracture 4

Avulsion of part of the intercondylar eminence is characteristic of children, whose anterior cruciate ligaments are stronger than the cartilage to which they are attached. Although it might be thought that full extension would tend to press the fragment down, any such tendency is opposed by the fact that full extension makes the anterior cruciate ligament taut. It is suggested that if the knee can be extended nearly fully, persisting displacement of the fragment is not going to interfere with function, except perhaps at the highest level of performance; in practice, this appears to be so.

Fracture 5

The tendon of the patella is stronger than the tongue-like epiphysis to which it is attached; if the fragment is tilted up as far as to a right angle it may press dangerously hard on the under surface of the skin. Being near the surface, it may be replaced by pressure over it although the fringe of soft tissue attached to its distal edge is likely to prevent it from being pushed fully home.

Fracture 6

Fracture-separation of the main epiphysis at the head of the tibia is rare and is usually the result of hyperextension force. Even at the moment of injury, when the displacement is greatest, the popliteal artery is unlikely to be injured by the back edge of the distal fragment.

Injuries of ligaments

Generally speaking, the collateral ligaments are injured when the knee is straight and the cruciate ligaments when it is bent. These injuries occur in young adults, whose bones withstand the stresses better than do their ligaments.

Collateral ligaments

Many of these injuries occur on sports fields, where the knee is bent sideways by another person either falling on to it or striking it in the course of a charge or a tackle. Alternatively, a sudden change of direction can catch the muscles off guard, with the result that the bones are momentarily out of control and move abnormally; this allows the energy to be applied to the ligaments instead of being absorbed by the muscles.

According to the direction of the injuring force, and how and where the limb is supported, the knee can be forced into valgus or varus or the femur can be driven backwards or forwards off the tibia or vice versa. Anteroposterior dislocations may leave the collateral soft tissues in sufficient continuity that once the joint has been replaced it is stable from side to side. The most dangerous complication is damage to the popliteal artery, particularly when the tibia is displaced backwards, but this is now amenable to surgical reconstruction.

Injuries of the collateral ligaments range from tearing of a few fibres at the joint line (Figure 11.2) to disruption of the capsule and ligaments for about half the circumference of the limb, in which case one or both cruciate ligaments are also torn. Successful repair requires adequate exposure of all the torn tissues and it should be mentioned that the lower end of the medial ligament has extensive attachment to the tibia deep to the tendons of sartorius, gracilis and semitendinosus, and can be likened to a hand that has been drawn out of a pocket and lies distorted near its mouth and perhaps on its outer surface. It needs to be replaced accurately and deeply within the pocket.

The lateral ligament is a simpler, cord-like structure that usually pulls bone from the femur or the head of the fibula when it gives way. Although the common peroneal nerve is not far away, it usually escapes injury unless there has been marked varus deformity. Repair of this ligament is usually easy but it is still necessary to use an exposure that will give access to all the torn structures on the lateral side of the joint.

Sprains of the collateral ligaments may accompany tears of the menisci and the combination of a history of twisting the knee under load, giving way with pain, and subsequent tenderness and swelling on the joint line and an effusion into the joint, may leave the precise diagnosis in doubt without the aid of arthroscopy.

Cruciate ligaments

There are important differences between ruptures of the anterior and those of the posterior ligament.

Anterior cruciate ligament

The ligament becomes taut when the knee is straight and it is responsible for the 'screw-home' movement of medial rotation of the femur on the tibia at the end of normal extension. Rupture can thus result from hyperextension. It can also result from full extension if the femur and tibia are separated as by a loose body or a displaced meniscus. When this happens, the ligament becomes taut before extension has been completed (see page 97) but it may be stretched rather than torn right through. Complete rupture is an inevitable consequence of injuries that cause complete rupture of either collateral ligament, because if the knee is straight the anterior cruciate ligament is taut and either adduction or abduction of the tibia on the femur will rupture it.

Posterior cruciate ligament

This ligament is taut when the knee is fully flexed but, like the anterior ligament, it is liable to be torn when the straight knee is forced into valgus or varus. It can also be torn if the tibia is forced backwards on the femur when the knee is flexed, as may happen in car crashes (Figure 4.4), falls, or from heavy blows on the sports field. There may therefore be a mark of impact on the front of the head of the tibia and, when the knees are flexed to right angles or a little beyond and the feet are firmly placed, the injured side shows obvious backward sagging (Figure 11.6a).

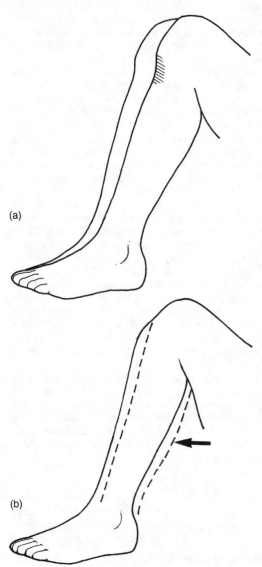

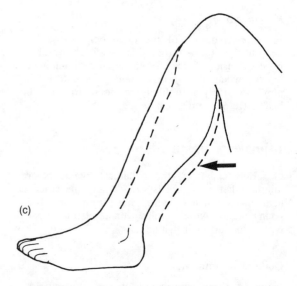

Figure 11.6. a, Backward sagging of the tibia resulting from rupture of the posterior cruciate ligament. The shading shows where there may be a mark of impact. b, The effect of pulling the leg forwards when the anterior cruciate ligament has been torn. c, The effect of pulling the leg forwards when the posterior cruciate ligament has been torn. The dotted lines represent the resting positions

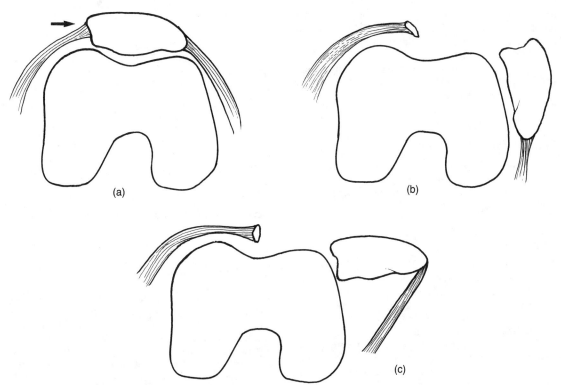

Figure 11.7. The cruciate ligaments: a, back view of the left knee; b, front view of the bent left knee. A, anterior; P, posterior

Draw sign. Although clinical and operative experience shows that rupture of a cruciate ligament can be present without there being increased anteroposterior movement of the flexed tibia on the femur, when it is possible this (draw) sign is evidence of rupture, or at least laxity, of one or other cruciate ligament. However, this sign can be misinterpreted unless it is remembered that when the anterior cruciate ligament has been torn the flexed tibia can be pulled forwards out of position (Figure 11.6b), whereas when the posterior ligament has been torn it can be pulled forwards into position (Figure 11.6c).

The cruciate ligaments are torn from bone and are not amenable to direct suture. It needs to be remembered that these ligaments are not rounded cords but have extensive attachments to both the tibia and the femur (Figure 11.7) and that both these attachments need to be restored as accurately as possible.

Patella

Dislocation of the patella is either the result of inborn structural abnormality that favours lateral displacement or it is the result of a blow.

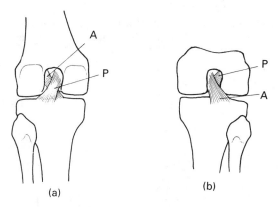

Figure 11.8. The two sorts of lateral dislocation of the patella

Lateral dislocation

A blow on its medial edge can drive the patella off the femur (Figure 11.8a). It usually lies with its articular surface against the lateral condyle of the femur (Figure 11.8b) but occasionally it sticks out sideways like a shelf (Figure 11.8c). In the former instance the knee is flexed and when it is straightened the patella returns to its proper position; in the latter instance the knee is straight but the patella is easily replaced by medially directed pressure. In either case, replacement is sometimes possible without anaesthesia.

Dislocation resulting from either existing structural defect or a blow can recur because of laxity on the medial side, where there may be chip fractures (Figure 11.3c).

Intra-articular dislocation

A blow on the upper pole of the patella can drive in downwards into the joint (Figure 11.9). The muscles stretch sufficiently for the extensor apparatus to remain functionally intact.

Rotary dislocation

A blow allegedly on the outer side of a soccer player's knee twisted the patella 90 degrees about a vertical axis so that its lateral edge was directed forwards (Colville, 1970). If the account of the injury was correct, the blow was presumably directed forwards on the outer edge of the patella (Figure 11.10). A blow directed posteromedially against the medial edge might have a similar effect, which would be facilitated if the knee were straight with the quadriceps relaxed.

Superior dislocation

The patella has been known to be locked above the articular surface of the femur by marginal osteophytes (Siegel and Mac, 1982).

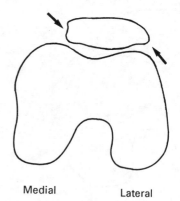

Medial   Lateral

Figure 11.10. Possible causes of rotary dislocation of the patella

Internal derangement of the knee

The typical history is of a twist or wrench that causes pain, giving way, perhaps a click and locking, and an effusion. This sequence can be the result of a torn meniscus, with or without torn ligaments, dislocation of the patella, osteochondral fracture or other cause of a loose body, or even chondromalacia of the patella. The distinction is made by means of a detailed history and examination, radiography and, if necessary, arthroscopy. In taking the history it is important to be aware that, although many patients complain that the knee locks, they do not usually mean that there was a sudden loss of the ability to extend the knee fully, i.e. true locking.

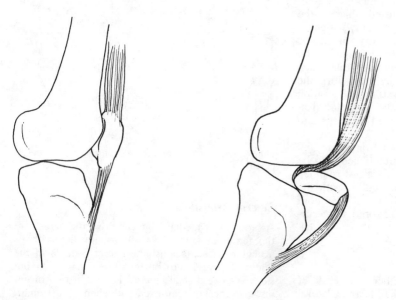

Figure 11.9. Intra-articular dislocation of the patella

Tears of the menisci

If the muscles are momentarily relaxed and caught off guard when the knee is bent and under load, the femur can slide sideways across the head of the tibia. For convenience, the head of the tibia is regarded as the fixed component of the joint. The knee gives way and is often said to have 'gone out'. This causes a momentary feeling of disconnection of the knee and a useful test is to ask the victim if for one ghastly moment it felt as though the leg had come off at the knee; the response is usually either a puzzled expression or a prompt agreement.

In the course of this sort of abnormal movement, one or other meniscus can be trapped and crushed between the femur and the tibia. The site and extent of any resulting tear (Figure 11.11) is presumably determined by the angle of the knee and the amount and direction of displacement of the femur on the tibia. When true locking occurs it is because part of the meniscus, usually the bucket handle, is displaced and holds the two bones slightly apart. In such cases the loss of extension persists in spite of full relaxation under general anaesthesia until it is corrected by manipulation. In some cases, however, the knee goes fully straight as the muscles relax and there is no click or jerk. This may be because of an effusion that makes the capsule and ligaments uncomfortably tense before the position of full extension is reached, but in some cases, especially when there is little or no effusion, the explanation may lie in damage to ligaments. Anything that separates the femur and the tibia, even momentarily, will cause the ligaments to become taut before the position in which this would normally happen is reached. If movement goes beyond that point, some ligaments will be injured. If they are only sprained, they will swell and consequently lose some of their extensibility. When this happens, even though the femur

and tibia are in normal contact and position, the ligaments will become taut short of full extension and in a conscious person this may be sufficient to induce protective muscular action; under anaesthesia this protective action is lost and the knee goes fully straight under the influence of gravity alone.

The ligaments most often injured in this way are the anterior cruciate, the deep fibres of the medial ligament and the adjoining coronary ligament attached to the periphery of the meniscus (Figure 11.11); hence the tenderness on the joint line.

Sometimes locking of a knee ceases spontaneously because the bucket-handle tear has been enlarged so much that the handle is pushed out of the way and the condyle of the femur moves unhampered in the gap.

McMurray's test is an attempt to trap a torn part of a meniscus momentarily between the tibia and the femur and the various tests of stability aim to show which ligaments are defective.

Chondromalacia patellae

This condition has been included because its clinical picture can be mistaken for that of more familiar derangements of the knee. Although the usual cause of damage to the articular surface is a blow on the patella, this bone can also be forced hard against the femur by muscular action in the course of twisting or wrenching the knee under load. Furthermore, as movement takes the roughened and softened area on the patella into the compressive load-bearing position on the femur, it allows the patella to move slightly towards the femur. Even this effective lengthening of the quadriceps is sufficient to impair its action. Softening on the femur can have a similar effect. These events can be compared with the passage of a wheel over a pothole in the road. The patient may have a momentary feeling of insecurity of the knee or the knee may give way and there is sometimes a feeling of sticking, which is referred to as locking; there may be a click or a crunch at the same time.

Wounds of the knee

Penetrating wounds

Pricks and punctures

Any wound near the knee may have entered it and the presence of an effusion into the joint should heighten suspicion that this has occurred.

Gunshot wounds

Low-velocity missiles can traverse the popliteal fossa and leave the neurovascular bundle passing

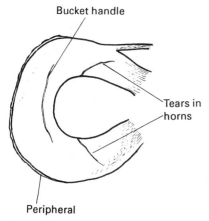

Bucket handle

Tears in horns

Peripheral

Figure 11.11. Sites of tears of menisci

unharmed across the gap, because the pliable soft tissues allow it to be pushed aside as the missile passes and then return to its normal position. So-called knee-capping is, in fact, a form of punishment by shooting the back of the knee or thigh with a pistol and may do little serious damage. High-velocity missiles would cause extensive damage such as might lead to amputation.

Flaying

If a pneumatic tyre passes over the knee, the skin is likely to be badly crushed against the bony prominences in the process of being split and torn in the usual way; the bony prominences and their attached muscles may be severely abraded.

References

Colville, J. (1970) An unusual case of intra-articular dislocation of the patella. *Injury*, **9**, 321

Siegel, M. G. and Mac, S. S. (1982) Superior dislocation of the patella with interlocking osteophytes. *Journal of Trauma*, **22**, 253

12

The leg

Fractures of the tibia and fibula

Acute fractures

Little needs to be said about acute fractures of the tibia. Spiral fractures usually follow simple falls and comminuted fractures result from the greater forces of heavy falls and road accidents. Although many fractures of the shaft of the tibia carry a high risk of delayed or non-union, the worst complications arise from damage to the soft tissues, and not only the skin.

As in the forearm, children's fractures may have hinges and respond to manipulation as described in Chapter 5 (page 38).

Neck of the fibula

In spite of its close relationship to this part of the fibula, the common peroneal nerve is only rarely injured by fractures there, which may accompany almost any fracture of the tibia.

Abduction of the upper end of the fibula

It is not very unusual to see widening of the gap between the upper ends of the tibia and fibula. In most cases no particular harm comes of it, but the combination should not be dismissed out of hand because it is sometimes associated with damage to the anterior tibial artery and consequent ischaemia of the extensor muscles in the leg. Failure to recognize this has, in my own experience, led to gas gangrene on the one hand and late breakdown of a wound following colliquative necrosis of the muscles on the other.

Dislocation of the head of the fibula

As a closed injury, this is rare and occurs when the leg is twisted and doubled up under its owner, as may happen at the bottom of a loose rugby scrum, for example. The head of the fibula is more often displaced forwards than backwards; in the latter case it may injure the common peroneal nerve. The dislocation is the result of a combination of proximal displacement of the fibula with lateral rotation and perhaps an element of rotation about a horizontal axis that takes the head either backwards or forwards. These forces could be applied by the foot if it were abducted and laterally rotated in the ankle mortice.

Open dislocation is likely to be part of a severe injury with accompanying damage to the anterior tibial artery and the common peroneal nerve.

Slow fractures

Apart from the familiar acute fractures, the leg is the commonest site of slow fractures in young adults. They result from repeated deflection in the course of powerful muscular action by male ballet dancers, military recruits and footballers.

Male ballet dancers

The fractures are high in the shaft of the tibia between the opposed forces applied from below when landing from a high leap and from above by the quadriceps in ensuring a soft landing on the one hand and providing a powerful take-off for a high leap on the other.

Military recruits

Running on roads while wearing heavy kit over-stresses the lower part of the shaft of the tibia.

Footballers

When the ankle joint becomes fully extended, the broader front part of the talus comes between the malleoli and forces the lateral one outwards. This twists the fibula slightly outwards and it also causes it to slide upwards a little, but the damaging movement is medial bowing, the effects of which appear a few inches above the malleolus.

These are tension fractures caused by deflection and they first become recognizable in radiographs as fine cracks on the convex surface of the part of the bone affected. Later, rarefaction appears on either side of the crack. In this way they resemble the slow fractures of Paget's disease, which can occur in the tibia as well as in the femur, and if such fractures become complete they are transverse.

Old persons

In old persons, slow fractures occasionally occur where the tibia splays out above the medial malleolus. If the bone becomes weak enough the upper part subsides into the lower, mainly on the inner side.

Soft tissues

Skin

Because the tibia is so close to the skin, blows directly over it may do damage to the skin in addition to the injuries from within by the bone or from without by other influences. Thus, what may at first appear to be a grade 1 open fracture with only a small wound, may be more severe because of grazing or crushing of the skin, with stripping or splitting of the fat beneath it. This can be recognized by touch: from without there is a soft-centred bruise or a graze and if the wound will admit a finger this will feel that there is no more than skin between it and the thumb outside. If information of this nature is not obtained or is ignored, conventionally placed incisions to expose the internal damage may cut off any blood supply that remains to the skin between the incision and the demonstrable damage. In such cases the surgeon should consider the practicability of making his incision through the damaged part, even though it might be necessary to make it longer than would otherwise be required to give adequate exposure. Even dead skin can be sewn up to give a germproof layer and if it remains dry and healthy, as it not infrequently does, there is no urgency about replacing it with skin grafts.

Flaying

This type of injury occurs more often in the leg than elsewhere and it can be so extensive that most of the skin hangs loose like a trouser leg that has been split lengthways. Occasionally, although widely stripped from the deeper tissues and badly crushed or bruised, the skin is unbroken and is distended by haematoma.

Bruises and blisters

Tense swelling can of itself cause the skin to blister. When there is an obvious haematoma this should be evacuated without delay so as to relieve the dangerous tension in the skin; however, if there is no obvious haematoma the blisters are sometimes an outward sign of Volkmann's ischaemia, for which prompt and extensive decompression by fasciotomy is urgently required.

Injuries of muscles

Large forces applied to the tibia inevitably cause more or less damage to the adjoining muscles, but there are two examples of this that deserve mention. The first is separation of the upper ends of the tibia and fibula, which has been dealt with on page 99; the second is direct crushing.

Crush injuries

A heavy blow may appear to have done no more than inflict a small wound over a mild fracture of the fibula, but if there is muscle between the site and the impact and the tibia it can be crushed through. A valuable warning to this effect is the presence of air bubbles as shown by radiographs made shortly after the injury. When they are small and close to the wound, air bubbles in the tissues are not likely to be of serious significance, but if they are some way from the wound in the skin they provide clear evidence that damage within the limb extends at least that far from the wound and should be explored.

Rupture of muscles and tendons

This type of injury is well known in the leg and usually occurs either at the lower end of the medial belly of the gastrocnemius or just above the point of the heel. Both result from violent effort and occur both in persons that are young and active and in those that are neither.

Torn muscle. There is sufficient bleeding within the deep fascia to cause tense and painful swelling of the calf that can mask the characteristic local tenderness. If at first there is some doubt about the diagnosis, suspicions should be aroused (or re-aroused) by the appearance of bruising on the inner side of the ankle, whither it tracks a few days later.

Rupture of the Achilles tendon. Occasionally the tendon is pulled from the calcaneus with more or less bone, but rupture usually occurs an inch or so above the bone. Retraction is often sufficient to cause a palpable if not a visible gap, but if the frayed ends are not pulled apart there is no gap but a palpable thickening at the site of injury. This, and the ability to flex the ankle, may prompt a diagnosis of partial rupture unless it is known that any muscle passing behind the ankle and into the foot can flex the ankle and unless the calf is gently squeezed. When this is done with the ankle free to move there is a slight but definite movement of flexion at the ankle; this is Thompson's test. If the foot does not move, gap or no, the tendon has been ruptured.

If partial rupture of the Achilles tendon does occur, it is rare.

Rupture of plantaris. If this injury occurs, it is rare. The muscle seems too small to rupture its tendon, which in my experience has always been intact when the Achilles tendon has been ruptured. If the muscle itself were torn, the signs and symptoms would be at the back of the knee joint, not lower in the calf.

Injuries of nerves and blood vessels

These are unusual except as part of severe injuries in which they are either torn by broken bone or crushed by external forces.

13

The ankle

Fractures and dislocations

It is still widespread practice to refer indiscriminately to fractures of the ankle as Pott's fractures. This is incorrect because Pott described a particular fracture-dislocation. Other patterns have acquired the names of Dupuytren, Wagstaffe and Maisonneuve, but eponymous titles tell us nothing of the forces that damage the ankle, understanding of which is necessary for successful treatment.

Most injuries of the ankle are caused by forces that are either transmitted through the foot or applied by the foot. An example of the former is a fall on to the heel that breaks the lower end of the tibia. Forces applied by the foot are most often the result of inversion of the foot. As the foot turns over on to its outer side it pulls on and may tear the lateral ligament of the ankle, but it can also have an apparently opposite effect that is usually referred to as a lateral rotation fracture of the fibula. The explanation for this apparent paradox lies in the phenomenon of torque conversion at the talocalcaneonavicular joint. Anatomically, this is a complicated joint, but Hicks (1953) showed that it functions as a hinge joint with an axis that is oblique to the X, Y and Z axes. When the foot swings inwards in the movement of inversion with the weight of the body on it, it applies an outwards twisting force to the talus and through it to the lateral malleolus.

Fractures of the ankle have been classified in painstaking detail according to the movements of the foot that generate the damaging forces (Lauge-Hansen, 1950) but a simpler classification is based on the patterns of injury that occur and the pulling and pushing forces that are directly responsible for them.

Lateral rotation injuries

Lateral rotation, which is often combined with translation, of the talus is the commonest injuring force and in adults it causes, by pushing and twisting, a spiral fracture of the fibula that starts at joint level and slopes upwards and backwards; occasionally the fracture occurs high in the shaft of the fibula. If this force pulls off the medial malleolus instead of tearing the ligament, it causes a transverse fracture below the level of the joint (Figure 13.1). In children these forces can cause fracture-separation of the lower ephiphysis of the tibia. Before the epiphysis fuses, separation may occur almost entirely through the epiphyseal line

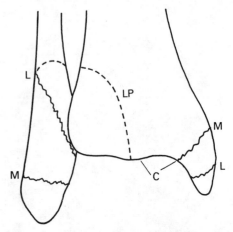

Figure 13.1. Patterns of fractures caused by rotation at the ankle. C, site of crushing in some cases; L, fractures caused by lateral rotation; LP, posterolateral fracture of the tibia; M, fractures caused by medial rotation or adduction

as a type 2 injury in Salter and Harris's classification (Salter and Harris, 1963). Alternatively, the fracture may be of Salter and Harris's type 3, with a vertical fissure through the epiphysis. In either case there is a shear piece at the posterolateral corner of the tibia. Fusion of the epiphysis starts on the medial side and spreads laterally, finishing at the anterolateral corner in the early teens. Before fusion is complete, the anterolateral corner is vulnerable to traction and may be pulled out as a block measuring one-half to three-quarters of an inch ($\approx$13–19 mm) along each side – Tillaux's fracture.

Rotation of the talus is accompanied by more or less displacement of it laterally and backwards; the amount of displacement can be classified as first degree, in which the talus remains in place, second degree, in which it is displaced laterally and third degree, in which it is displaced backwards as well. There are three possible effects: (1) rupture or avulsion of the anterior, inferior tibiofibular ligament. In adults little or no bone is pulled from the tibia but in the early teens Tillaux's fracture may occur; (2) rupture of the interosseous tibiofibular ligament with more or less separation of the two bones. (3) fracture of the posterolateral corner of the tibia (Figure 13.1, LP), which is sometimes referred to as though it were a third malleolus as in the description trimalleolar fracture-subluxation. This fragment remains firmly attached to the lateral malleolus by the posterior, inferior tibiofibular ligament with the result that the fragments move together. If the lateral malleolus is replaced accurately and fixed securely, the articular surface of the tibia is usually accurately restored. The posterior fragment is not often big enough to need to be fixed in order to withstand the forces applied to it by the talus. Closed manipulation may be less successful and may leave an unacceptable step.

The greater the degree of displacement, the more extensive is the tearing of the capsule and ligaments of the ankle and the greater the degree of instability of the joint.

There is an extreme form of this injury in which the foot may be rotated as much as 90 degrees and the upper fragment of the fibula becomes displaced behind the tibia and locked there, with the extensor tendons occupying the notch in which the fibula normally lies (Figure 13.2a). A milder variety of this injury leaves the foot pointing more nearly forwards (Figure 13.2b). If the nature of this type of injury is clearly understood, careful examination of the radiographic appearances (Figure 13.2c, d) will enable the lesion to be identified.

1. The talus is behind the tibia in the lateral view and overlaps it in the anteroposterior view.
2. The medial malleolus appears to be at the back edge of the tibia whereas its natural position is well forward. The explanation is that when the X-ray cassette is placed beside the foot for the lateral view of the ankle, there is enough lateral rotation of the foot to yield an oblique view of the ankle that displaces the shadow of the medial malleolus backwards.

With both degrees of displacement of the talus the extensor tendons occupy the notch for the fibula and the skin is stretched tightly over the front edge of the tibia.

If an attempt to correct this deformity is made in order to relieve the pressure on the skin, it will fail because the talus and the shaft of the fibula are jammed tightly behind the tibia. Even when the lesion is exposed surgically it may require considerable force to overcome the tension in the interosseous membrane and lever the fibula free from the tibia.

Open injuries

Severe displacement of the foot can split the skin and leave one or other malleolus sticking out.

Medial rotation injuries

When these occur, which is not often, they cause spiral fractures that extend upwards from the base of the medial malleolus and transverse fractures of the fibula below the horizontal joint line (Figure 13.1, M).

Abduction injuries

The lateral malleolus is pushed laterally and the fibula is broken by bending a few inches above the ankle. There is a shear piece on the lateral side. The lower end of the fibula may or may not be torn from the tibia. Any fracture of the medial malleolus is of the avulsion sort (Figure 13.3). This is the pattern of fracture illustrated by Pott in his description of the fracture that properly bears his name. Very rarely, the tibiofibular ligaments are torn without fracture and sometimes this allows the talus to come between the two bones. This sometimes happens when there has been a high fracture of the fibula.

Adduction injuries

When these injuries occur the pattern may not be distinguishable from that caused by medial rotation but sometimes there is crushing of the articular surface of the tibia at the base of the medial malleolus (Figure 13.1, C). If this happens before growth has ceased it can lead to serious deformity.

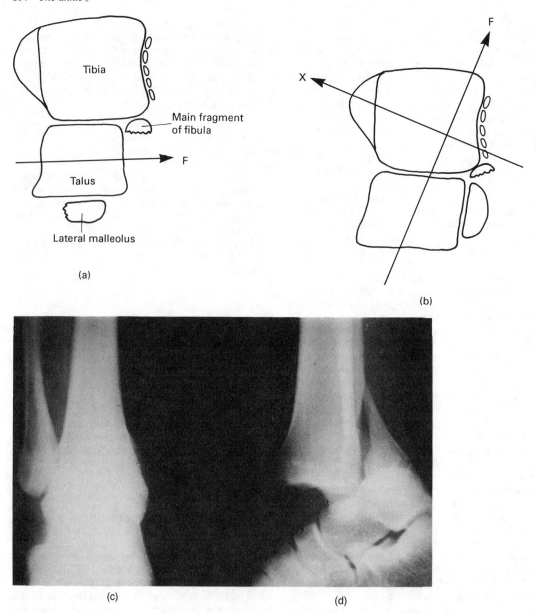

Figure 13.2. Dislocation of the talus with locking of the fibula. a, Plan view of the left ankle with the foot pointing sideways; b, as above but with the foot pointing nearly forwards; F, long axis of the foot; X, central x-ray; c and d, anteroposterior and lateral views of dislocation (b)

Burst fractures of the tibia

Occasionally the lower end of the tibia is comminuted by a blow applied directly beneath it and the fragments separate in both coronal and sagittal directions. More often, the talus slides forwards as well as being driven upwards and it shears off the front of the lower end of the tibia with more or less comminution.

Posterior translation of the talus

The main justification for including this variety of fracture-dislocation is that some patients give a clear account of catching the heel of a shoe on a step or ledge and falling forwards. Both malleoli are broken by being pushed apart by the broader front part of the body of the talus. Occasionally the back edge of the tibia is broken as well, but

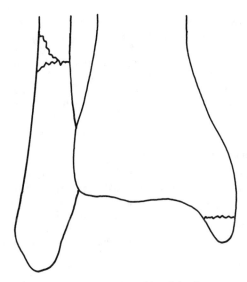

Figure 13.3. Fractures caused by abduction

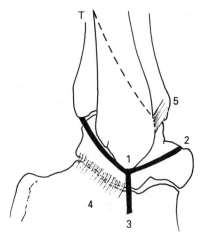

Figure 13.4. The ligaments on the outer side of the ankle. 1, Attachment of the lateral ligament to the fibula; 2, attachment of the anterior band of the lateral ligament to the talus; 3, calcaneofibular ligament; 4, posterior talocalcanean capsule; 5, anterior, inferior tibiofibular ligament; T, site of tenderness with an oblique fracture of the fibula; - - - -, line of oblique fracture of the fibula

there is nothing characteristic about the radiological pattern of the injury.

Dislocation of the ankle

Dislocation without fracture is very rare. The talus may move forwards or be tilted medially out of the mortice, or it may move upwards between the tibia and fibula after they have been separated.

Sprains at the ankle

These almost always follow inversion of the foot while it is under load. Stress falls first upon the anterior band of the lateral ligament, which tears at one or other end, where small avulsion fractures may occur (Figure 13.4, 1 and 2). Up to this point the talus tilts little or not at all on the tibia, but if the force continues to act and the talus begins to tilt, the middle band of the lateral ligament is torn. At the same time, the movement of inversion brings the calcaneus forwards under the talus and this results in tearing of the capsule of the posterior talocalcanean joint (Figure 13.4). The extreme deformity is either dislocation of the talus by medial tilting or talocalcanean (or abtalar) dislocation.

Tilting of the talus sometimes chips a flake off its superolateral corner. The resulting dome fracture resembles in appearance the osteochondral fracture of the medial condyle of the femur (fracture 2 in Figure 11.1).

If there is lateral rotation of the talus in the mortice, this tears the anterior, inferior tibiofibular ligament, with or without a sprain-fracture. When

this occurs there may also be tearing of the superior extensor retinaculum, as a result of which swelling spreads a few inches up the anterolateral aspect of the leg.

Inversion of the foot tightens the lateral part of the inferior extensor retinaculum, which is attached to the upper surface of the calcaneus (Figure 13.5) and may also be torn.

Apart from the capsule, the other ligaments of the ankle are only rarely injured without serious accompanying fractures.

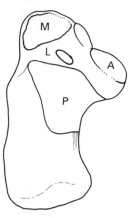

Figure 13.5. Upper surface of the left calcaneus. A, Anterior articular surface; L, site of attachment of the inferior extensor retinaculum; M, site of attachment of the extensor digitorum brevis; P, posterior articular surface

Swelling, tenderness and diagnosis

Immediately after injury, swelling and tenderness occur precisely at the site(s) of injury and may enable a careful examiner to make a confident and correct diagnosis. As swelling spreads, tenderness becomes more diffuse. Nevertheless, the attachments of ligaments and the malleoli should be palpated carefully. In addition, the back of the fibula should be palpated; both a sprain and an oblique fracture will cause tenderness and swelling in front but only an oblique fracture will cause tenderness at the back, 2–3 inches ($\approx$50–70 mm) above the tip of the malleolus (Figure 13.4, T). It should also be mentioned that the lateral side of the calcaneus and the base of the fifth metatarsal bone should be palpated.

Effusion into the ankle joint

This can sometimes be recognized as small bulges between the malleoli and the extensor tendons. Fluctuation may be demonstrated between them but they are soon masked by more general swelling. Effusion is a useful warning that fracture may have occurred and when an effusion is diagnosed it should prompt a particularly careful examination of radiographs.

Instability of the ankle

Complete rupture of the lateral ligament can be followed by repeated 'going over' of the ankle because the talus is free to tilt in its socket. Repeated going over can also occur with little or no tilting of the talus. The explanation may be that lesser tears of the ligament, and perhaps of the extensor retinaculum, on the outer side interfere with the proprioceptive impulses that initiate protective action by the muscles that can evert the foot.

Dislocation of the peroneal tendons

Occasionally, vigorous eversion of the foot, perhaps with extension of the ankle, causes the two peroneal tendons to jump from their groove behind and below the fibula and on to its lateral surface. Tearing or natural laxity of the retinaculum or a shallow groove are the most likely causes.

References

Hicks, J. H. (1953) The mechanics of the foot. *Journal of Anatomy,* **87**, 345

Lauge-Hansen, N. (1950) Fractures of the ankle II. Combined experimental–surgical and experimental–roentgenologic investigations. *Archives of Surgery,* **60**, 957

Salter, R. B. and Harris, W. R. (1963) Injuries of the epiphyseal plate. *Journal of Bone and Joint Surgery,* **45A**, 587

14

The foot

Fractures and dislocations

These injuries are caused by the twisting forces of inversion and eversion; by deflections such as abduction, adduction, flexion and extension; by crushing and by impact, including stubbing, which is end-on impact, and by traction. These forces may act in combination and most of them result from heavy falls and road accidents in which the floor of a vehicle is driven hard against the foot, which may also be trapped by the pedals. Classification based on the injuring force(s) is much more usefully informative than that based on anatomical descriptions of which bones and joints have been affected. Although the radiological appearances can be very confusing, experience enables one to resolve them into essentially simple patterns that are sometimes surprisingly easy to treat.

Twisting injuries

Inversion

As mentioned in Chapter 13, this force can displace the talus in the ankle mortice or the rest of the foot from the talus as talonavicular dislocation, in which case the head of the talus forms a prominent dorsilateral lump with the skin stretched tightly over it; sometimes the skin splits and leaves the under-surface of the talus exposed in the wound. If the two injuries are combined the result is total dislocation of the talus, which may lead to loss of the bone if the skin over it splits open.

A much milder inversion injury is avulsion of the base of the fifth metatarsal bone. Confusion between fracture and the epiphysis will be avoided if it is remembered that fractures are transverse and the epiphyseal line is longitudinal; occasionally both are present.

Eversion

This is a much rarer cause of injury than inversion and perhaps its most striking result is dislocation of the navicular bone downwards from the head of the talus. The tendon of the tibialis anterior is sometimes pulled between the head of the talus and the rest of the foot and has to be extracted surgically. A distinction between some injuries of this type and some of the severe abduction injuries (see page 108) may not be possible.

Injury by deflection

Adduction

Although the fore part of the foot can be pushed medially by a blow on its outer side, adduction injuries can also result from forcible stubbing or from end-to-end compression that accentuates the natural slight lateral bowing of the foot and so causes crushing on the medial side and traction on the lateral side of the foot. The most characteristic of these injuries is talonavicular fracture-subluxation in which the navicular bone moves medially on the head of the talus, is crushed against it and may indent the medial part of the head. There are sometimes accompanying fractures of the bases of the metatarsal bones (Figure 14.1). In the antero-posterior radiographic view the talonavicular injury may not be clearly shown; in the lateral view the navicular appears to have sustained a roughly horizontal fracture.

In spite of swelling it can be seen that the natural concavity of the foot has been accentuated

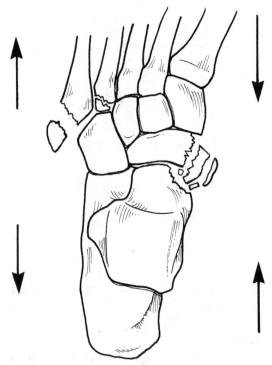

Figure 14.1. Talonavicular fracture-subluxation with fractures of metatarsal bones. The arrows indicate the directions of the forces that are responsible

and the skin on the inner side of the sole may be creased as a result of this.

Less often the force is concentrated on the tarsometatarsal joints, where crush fractures are more likely than dislocation, except of the first metatarsal bone.

Abduction

The damage is mostly at the tarsometatarsal joints. All five metatarsal bones may be displaced but quite often the first remains in place and the other four are shifted laterally, with numerous chip fractures at their bases. Characteristic radiological features are widening of the space between the first two metatarsal bones, loss of the tarsometatarsal joint spaces and displacement of the styloid process of the fifth metatarsal bone so that it comes near to the proximal edge of the cuboid bone. Although swelling will mask it to some extent, the discerning eye will recognize that the front part of the foot is inclined outwards.

A particularly dangerous but fortunately rare variety of this type of injury is accompanied by reversal of the natural concavity of the sole and tears the medial plantar artery and some of its branches. An injury of this sort might also result from a heavy weight falling on to the foot.

Occasionally the line of fracture passes through or between the cuneiform or the cuboid bones.

Extension

The most familiar and striking of these injuries affect the talus (Figure 14.2). In the mildest versions the impact of the front edge of the tibia on the upper surface of the neck of the talus causes a fracture there. The springy grip of the ankle mortice on the talus then causes the body of the bone to flex so that its narrower posterior part occupies the mortice. This means that if the foot is at a right angle to the leg, the head of the talus appears to be dorsally displaced on the neck. More serious injuries of this type show mild displacement of the body of the talus in relation to the calcaneus but the most severe injuries dislocate the body entirely. If the extension is extreme the tibia pushes the body of the talus out of joint and it follows a curved and twisting path over the facet of the calcaneus and finishes on the medial side of the calcaneus with its broken surface facing proximally and its upper surface facing medially. The skin and the posterior tibial neurovascular bundle are stretched over the displaced bone and the bundle is at risk from an incision to effect surgical correction. The medial ligament of the ankle joint may remain intact and provide a useful source of blood for the body of the talus.

Fracture-dislocations of intermediate severity also occur. These injuries used to be known as aviator's astragalus because they were caused by the upward thrust of the rudder bar of a crashing aeroplane.

If the foot can be pulled away from the leg it may be possible to push the body of the talus back into place between the tibia and the calcaneus but it will be flexed in the mortice; open correction and fixation is more reliable.

Flexion

Fracture of the middle of the foot by flexion is rare and is usually the result of great violence, the effect of which is aided by support for the posterior part of the foot as by the footrest of a motor bicycle. In such cases there is likely to be severe damage to the skin and the metatarsal bones. Closed injuries can also occur in which there is no characteristic pattern of the comminution in the tarsometatarsal region.

Instability after injury of the foot

Most of the injuries that have been described above cause so much instability that the only certain way of holding the foot in the right shape

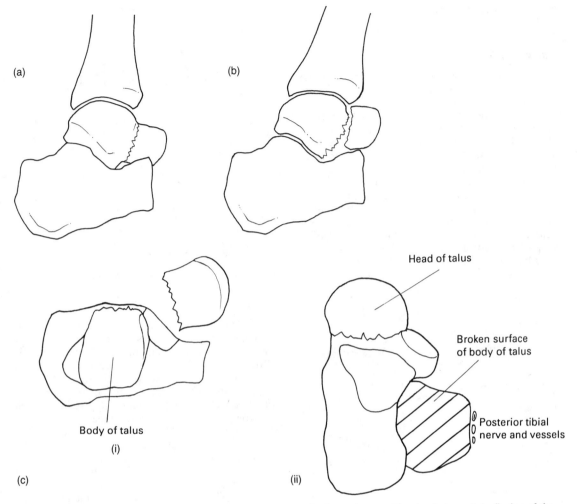

Figure 14.2. Fractures of the talus and displacement: a, a crack in the neck caused by simple impact; b, flexion of the body of the talus, often with mild subluxation; c, dislocation of the body of the talus (i) from medial side, (ii) from above

is by surgical fixation, but some talocalcaneonavicular dislocations are stable after correction. More or less stiffness of the foot is inevitable but in the absence of deformity it is not usually much of a handicap, whereas the combination of stiffness and deformity can be crippling.

Injury of the skin

Although the skin, particularly on the dorsum of the foot, may be injured by crushing or impact, it can also be damaged by being stretched over prominent and sometimes jagged bone beneath it. Whatever the cause, the presence of damaged skin may have to be taken into consideration when planning incisions or choosing between internal and external fixation.

Crushing and impact

A distinction between crushing and impact might be made on the basis of the speed or the duration of the application of the injuring force but in practice the words may be regarded as being synonymous. Crushing follows falls on to the heel, weights falling on the foot and end-to-end compression.

Falls injure the calcaneus or the talus.

Fracture of the talus

The body of the bone is sometimes caught fair and square between the tibia and the calcaneus and is squashed more or less severely. This sort of injury is rare and it causes marked stiffness that is the result of avascular necrosis and will be none the less for attempts at reconstruction of the bone.

Fracture of the calcaneus

Whether the force is applied from above in the course of a fall or from below by an explosion, the effect on the calcaneus is the same, although there are two radiologically distinct patterns of fracture (Figure 14.3). In both, the posterior articular facet is driven into the bone beneath but in one pattern there is a backward bony projection from the facet and in the other there is not. Otherwise, depending on the severity of the crushing force, there are more or less extensive fractures between the two articular facets on the calcaneus and of the lateral wall of the bone below the posterior facet. These occur because the blunt chisel-like front edge of the posterior articular facet of the talus is driven down into the calcaneus (Figure 14.4) and because of the accompanying descent of the articular facet

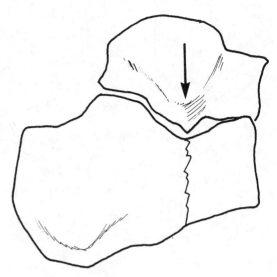

Figure 14.4. Chisel-like action of the talus under heavy load

and valgus inclination of the heel. The result is broadening and eversion of the heel, which is best seen from behind. Sometimes the deformity is sufficient for the calcaneus to press on the lateral malleolus or the tendons between them and cause trouble later. The concavity of the sole is obliterated first by deformity and later by swelling, which is accompanied by bruising that has tracked from the fracture and is characteristic of this injury.

Occasionally, a fall on to the heel breaks off the medial tuberosity of the calcaneus.

Most crushing injuries affect the toes, where they range from mere splits in the skin, perhaps with loosening of the nail, to open fractures of the phalanges with or without fractures of the necks of metatarsal bones. Unless they are very heavy, weights falling on the middle of the foot are likely to inflict more damage on the skin than on the skeleton, in which there is no characteristic pattern.

End-to-end compression

At its worst this causes talocalcaneal injuries of the sort shown by Figure 14.1 but lesser injuries can occur.

Fracture-subluxation of the first cuneometatarsal joint. This is homologous with Bennett's injury in the hand. A blow in the line of the first metatarsal bone causes its base to rear up on the dorsum of the foot, where the easily visible prominence effectively shortens the extensor hallucis longus and cocks the big toe up (Figure 14.5). This combination is characteristic.

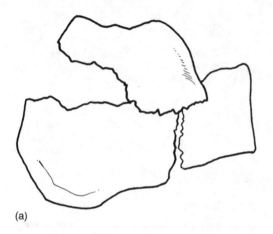

(a)

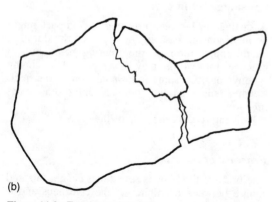

(b)

Figure 14.3. Fractures of the calcaneus: a, tongue type; b, simple depression type

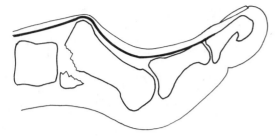

Figure 14.5. Pedal homologue of Bennett's fracture-subluxation

Metatarsocuboid injuries. A similar injury to the last sometimes affects the fourth and fifth metatarsal bones, whose joints with the cuboid are quite steeply inclined and so allow proximal displacement, usually with small fractures of the metatarsal or cuboid bones. Occasionally, a fairly thick flake is split off the side of the cuboid bone (Figure 14.6).

Fractures of the necks of metatarsal bones. Violent stubbing can break the necks of one or more of the four lateral metatarsal bones and there may also be injuries at their bases.

As in the hand, the amount of deformity of fractures of the metatarsal bones may be underestimated if anteroposterior and oblique radiographic views are accepted; true lateral views of the broken bones should be insisted on. This is of particular importance in the case of the first metatarsal because uncorrected extension deformity of this bone will cause the foot to roll into valgus

enough to bring the ball of the big toe back on to the ground. This can cause considerable discomfort, especially in an elderly person's foot.

Fracture-subluxation of the big toe. Violent stubbing can crush the base of the proximal phalanx and shift the bone proximally on the head of the metatarsal.

Tuberosity of the navicular bone. This is sometimes large and exists as a separate bone, which can be mistaken for a fracture when a blow causes pain, swelling and tenderness over it.

Sesamoid bones of the big toe. These are quite often in two or three pieces but they are rarely broken.

Avulsion fractures

Most of these are sprain-fractures of the base of the fifth metatarsal bone, of the neck of the talus, of the anterior process of the calcaneus and of the cuboid bone.

Calcaneus

The so-called beak fracture of the calcaneus occurs usually in elderly persons, whose bones are weaker than their Achilles tendons. It is an avulsion fracture and the back edge sometimes presses dangerously hard on the under-surface of the skin.

Slow fractures

The most familiar is the march fracture of the second metatarsal bone and it sometimes happens that, once the head of the second ceases to take its full share of weight, the load is transferred to the third and it later gives way. Occasionally, fast bowlers overstress the shaft of the fifth metatarsal bone and cause it to give way.

Although it occurs slowly, the fragmentation of the head of the second metatarsal bone in Freiburg's disease and of the navicular bone in Köhler's disease is not the result of overstressing a normal bone but of a degenerative process.

Dislocation of the toes

These are almost always dorsal. When multiple, they are usually the result of falls or road accidents but a single toe is often dislocated by stubbing a bare foot. Dorsal dislocation of the big toe may cause flexion of the interphalangeal joint because the long flexor tendon is effectively shortened as it passes round the head of the metatarsal bone. This flexion distinguishes the cocking up of the toe from that shown in Figure 14.5.

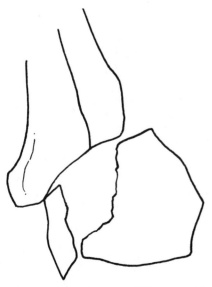

Figure 14.6. Metatarsocuboid fracture-subluxation

Flaying of the foot

Unless it is protected by stout footwear, a foot that is run over may suffer such severe damage to the skin that it is split and stripped from most of the foot. Fortunately, the skin under the heel is usually spared and this alone may enable the patient to lead an active life in spite of having most of the foot covered with split skin grafts.

Flaying may destroy some toes. Apparently less severe injuries occur in which the splits in the skin are smaller but there can still be extensive undermining, with the consequent need for skin grafting.

If a wheel is hard rather than having a pneumatic tyre, the damage to the bones, joints and tendons as well as the skin can be severe enough to result in amputation.

15

Injuries of soft tissues

So far, the soft tissues have been considered mainly as components of the more severely disruptive injuries, but it may be helpful to draw this scattered information together and combine it with a more general account of injuries of a less disruptive nature that affect the soft tissues.

Definitions of terms

Closed injuries

These are the result of impact, crushing or traction. The distinction between impact and crushing is to some extent artificial because it depends mainly on the duration of the injuring force and on the amount of 'follow through'.

Open injuries

The skin may be breached from within or from without; the difference is important because the risk of infection is usually greater with inwardly than with outwardly penetrating injuries. Furthermore, the wounds may be tidy, as when made by sharp objects, or untidy as when made by blunt or rough objects or by missiles travelling at high velocity.

Loose connective tissues

In all injuries of soft tissues the loose connective tissues play a very important part. This applies particularly to the connective tissues that separate one structure from another but also to those that exist within the structures themselves. They are planes of cleavage that are torn open by the injuring forces and inevitably take part in the disruption of most anatomical structures. This is seen most clearly and dramatically in a limb that has been run over and has had its skin torn loose and split. The exposed muscles have been separated and more or less damaged and the main neurovascular bundles are often dissected out in a similar manner. In other cases, the connective tissues confer what may be a protective mobility, on neurovascular bundles in particular, with the result that they may be displaced by a penetrating object and then return to cross, perhaps undamaged, a gap in the tissues.

Slowly travelling missiles and other penetrating objects may be diverted along planes of cleavage rather than continuing on their previous course. Similarly, loose connective tissues may allow broken bones to emerge between muscles rather than tearing through them.

Any structure that is divided, by whatever means, shows some tendency to retract and it does so within a more or less well-defined sheath. Crushing causes serious and more or less extensive disruption of tissues that may make identification difficult, whereas a clean cut disturbs the natural relationships of the divided structures little or not at all. For this reason, the surgeon exploring such a wound in search for, and identification of, nerves, blood vessels, muscles and tendons, will be well advised to try to avoid disturbing those relationships by formal dissection and to rely as far as possible on the careful use of retractors and forceps, aided if necessary by cross-sectional diagrams of the part. There is no shame in sending for a text book of anatomy. Careful inspection in a good light will often enable a knowing eye to recognize the faint traces of blood that lie in the wake of retracted structures.

For similar reasons, when a surgeon has followed a penetrating wound through one layer he must examine the next layer carefully in search of penetration that may be some way away from the track that he has already found. To do this it may suffice to retract the existing track carefully in all directions or it may be necessary to enlarge it. As each new layer is encountered it must be examined in a similar manner until the end of the track has been established beyond doubt. If this proves to be inside a joint or one of the cavities of the trunk it may be advisable to explore the cavity through a separate, formal exploratory incision rather than by enlarging the wound.

Skin and fat

Skin

Closed injuries

These are mostly the result of superficial burns and crushing. Where skin is crushed close over bone it sometimes looks brown and translucent like waxed paper and the superficial vessels may look like black streaks. Prolonged crushing under the weight of an unconscious body renders the skin thin and pale but once the pressure is relieved it swells and blisters and acquires an ill-defined red margin of variable extent. In this respect it soon comes to look like a burn but, unlike a burn, the muscle beneath it is liable to swell and may require decompression in order to prevent Volkmann's ischaemia.

The skin is occasionally damaged from within by the pressure of displaced bone, by contact with broken bone or by stretching. Undamaged skin is remarkably tolerant of stretching but, if it has been damaged and is then stretched, skin may show blistering. This can happen when a blow causes marked swelling, as by an haematoma; the occurrence of blistering in such a case is valuable warning that decompression is required.

Stretching and blistering may also occur in cases of Volkmann's ischaemia.

Open injuries

There is little to add to what has appeared in previous chapters but the following points are worth repeating.

1. The elasticity of skin can allow quite large foreign bodies to enter through what appear to be small holes.
2. Wounds of entry made by high-velocity missiles are often small and may be neat, whereas those of exit are larger and ragged.
3. The possibility that all wounds over joints and the cavities of the trunk have entered them requires serious consideration.
4. The tracks of wounds penetrating several layers of tissue may be broken up when the victim's posture is altered after wounding.
5. Tendons exposed in wounds must be seen to move through their full excursion before they are declared to be uninjured.
6. Wounds made from within by spikes of bone may be accompanied by serious and perhaps extensive damage to the under-surface of the skin that causes soft-centred bruising.
7. Incisions made close to damaged areas of skin may cut off the blood supply of the intervening skin.
8. Skin that has been torn loose when a part has been run over by a rubber tyre is usually accompanied by any subcutaneous fat, to which it is firmly connected.

Fat

Apart from penetrating injuries, fat may be split by impact or by shearing. In the former case the split is roughly perpendicular to the surface (Figure 15.1a); in the latter it is roughly parallel to the surface. Shearing injuries may occur within the substance of the fat or between it and the subjacent tissues, where there is a well-defined plane of cleavage. This can be regarded as closed flaying. Although the skin may be unbroken at the time of injury, it may be doomed from the start because of crushing and stretching, to which is often added the further stretching caused by accumulated blood (Figure 15.1b). In such cases, decompression may allow some of the stripped skin to survive; if this is to be undertaken, the necessary – and generous – incision should be made through the worst-damaged skin, which it may be possible to identify by feel as having been detached from the fat beneath. If such skin is pinched between a finger and thumb it is easy to recognize the fact that there is no more than two layers of skin between the digits (Figure 15.1c). The area may well show bruising and grazing as well. Attempts to evacuate subcutaneous haematomata by even multiple suction drains are not usually successful.

Muscles, tendons and ligaments

Muscles

Closed injuries

Crushing most often occurs with fractures, the damage being done by the force that breaks the bone, by the broken bone or by both. Less violent impact can crush through a muscle where it is close to bone and this is an important cause of soft-centred bruises. To the eye, the part is swollen and discoloured but to the finger it is obvious

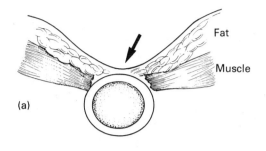

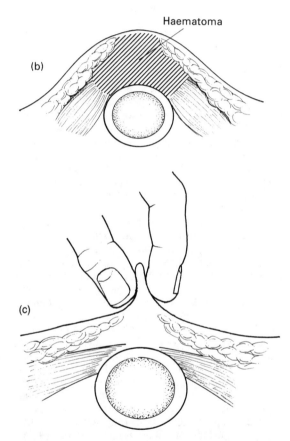

Figure 15.1. a, Muscle and fat are crushed against bone; b, a soft-centred bruise forms in the gap; c, the unpadded skin can be recognized as such when it is picked up between finger and thumb

that the skin can be pushed in until it reaches bone.

Crushing can also strip muscle from its bony attachment and may then force it out through a break in the skin, as described in Chapter 7.

Traction. Muscles can be torn by sudden and powerful action against perhaps unexpected resistance and also by slow stretching and sudden pulls

when they are contracting. Sometimes the tearing takes place within the substance of the muscle. If the sheath of the muscle remains intact the appearance may suggest no more than bruising within it, but if the sheath is opened in such cases it will be found that the torn ends of the muscle are separated by blood clot. That this has happened may also be suggested by redundancy of tendons. In other cases the tendon may be torn from the belly of the muscle. This seems to be more likely when the junction between the tissues is oblique rather than transverse.

Nerves and blood vessels supplying muscles. Any injury will do some damage to these sources of supply but in most cases it requires no more than the removal of the damaged part of the muscle. In some cases, particularly when there is a well-defined neurovascular hilum (Brash, 1955), crushing, avulsion or cutting may separate this from the muscle that it supplies. Although it may be technically possible to repair the structures, I have on numerous occasions been struck by the excellent function that follows the loss of large amounts of muscle, even the complete removal of, for example, the flexor digitorum superficialis. It is perhaps fair to state that there is only one place for dead meat – the bucket.

Ischaemia of muscle. It is here necessary to say no more than that whenever muscle becomes swollen within an unyielding compartment, for whatever reason, it should be completely decompressed by means of extensive fasciotomy and at the earliest opportunity.

Heart

In some respects the heart can be regarded as a solid organ but it does have sufficient of the characteristics of muscle to be considered here.

Closed injuries. A blow over the heart may cause contusion of the myocardium of more or less severity. Occasionally it causes thrombosis of a coronary artery, particularly if it is already affected by atherosclerosis.

During systole the heart is remarkably tough but during diastole it is more vulnerable, especially by crushing forces, among which must now be included external compression by resuscitators. These injuries range from bruising of the myocardium to more or less extensive tears of the walls, septa, valves or their retaining bands.

Open injuries. The heart is the obvious target for many assailants. Small wounds may seal themselves and heal without treatment; others leak into the pericardium and cause tamponade. Aspiration may relieve this but exploration and formal repair are usually necessary to prevent recurrence. Damage to coronary vessels, septa and valves are now amenable to repair if the patient reaches hospital alive and can be resuscitated.

Tendons

Closed injuries

Crushing forces may strip tendons from their bony attachments; otherwise, their toughness, resilience and, in some places, their lateral mobility, enable them to resist most forces of this sort.

Avulsion tends to uproot bone in young persons but to tear the tendon itself in older ones. The end of a tendon of the flexor digitorum profundus may retract as far as the palm but if it has bone attached this may jam in the decussation of the flexor digitorum superficialis and interfere with its function.

Attrition and rupture. Rheumatoid arthritis is a well-known cause of degeneration of tendons, to which may be added the effects of sharp edges or spikes of bone. Delayed rupture of the tendon of the extensor pollicis longus at the wrist after fracture is presumably caused by degenerative change, although there is no clear explanation of how and why this occurs. The subject has been considered in more detail in Chapter 5.

Dislocation. Degenerative diseases may allow tendons gradually to slide out of place. In the hand, a blow or a cut sometimes divides the lateral connection and allows an extensor tendon to dislocate at once. Otherwise, dislocation is the result of distortion or displacement that allows a tendon to tear or stretch its retaining structure, as in the shoulder and at the ankle.

Open injuries

Unlike muscles, tendons are much more often cut than injured by closed means. It is perhaps worth repeating that whenever a tendon is seen in a wound it should be made to move through its full excursion before being declared to be uninjured.

Ligaments

Ligaments may be scraped or ground away from their attachments to bone. They are most often injured by traction in the course of sprains and dislocations, in which they are almost always torn from bone, often with some bone, rather than through their substance. They may then become tucked into the joint concerned or otherwise displaced and in need of surgical replacement and repair.

Solid organs

In general, moderate impact causes a more or less clean split whereas larger forces and crushing increase the size of the split, which also becomes more complex, with branches running in several directions, and is accompanied by pulping and perhaps separation of part(s) of the organ. Bleeding may be severe because main blood vessels are liable to be torn. Open injuries are for all practical purposes caused from without.

Different organs behave in different ways and deserve individual consideration.

Brain

Closed injuries

Most of these result from a blow on the head but, unless there is a depressed fracture of the skull, the damaged parts of the brain are not only at the site of impact but also where inertia brings the brain into forcible contact with bony ridges and other prominences or with the dural partitions. This occurs when the head is free to move on, as well as with, the neck and because the skull and the brain are for the most part not in contact. If the head is not free to move on impact, damage to the brain requires much more energy, sufficient to cause serious deformation of the skull.

If the head is struck when it is free to move, it twists and tilts on the neck on one or more of the X, Y and Z axes. These movements are rotational accelerations (Pudenz and Sheldon, 1946). When the head is struck, the skull is set in motion before the brain, which means that in the area of impact the skull is driven against the brain, whereas at the opposite pole, or end of the curved path of acceleration, the skull moves away from the brain. Depending upon the amount of energy that is transferred, this separation of skull from brain can be sufficient to result in what can reasonably be regarded as explosive decompression. High-speed cinematography shows that fragments can spurt from the surface of the brain (Gurdjian, 1971). These are the well-known coup and contrecoup lesions, which range from mild bruising to extensive pulping, with more or less extensive subarachnoid bleeding.

Similar reactions occur between the brain and the dural partitions, which have smooth, flat surfaces that are not rigid and cause correspondingly less damage unless the impact is against the edge of a partition.

The role of accelerational forces was well shown by Holbourn (1945), who calculated from the physical characteristics of the brain and the skull, the degree and extent of damage to the brain resulting from blows on the head. The results of his calculations closely resembled the findings familiar to pathologists.

At the same time, the sudden acceleration and, no less, the sudden deceleration that results when a swiftly moving head is brought sharply to a halt sets up shearing stresses within the substance of the brain (Strich, 1961) and in the brain stem, which can undergo very rapid but striking deformation as a result of a blow on the head (Gurdjian, 1971), Until the damage to neural fibres was demonstrated histologically, the sometimes normal appearance of the brain post mortem allowed numerous and fanciful explanations of the cause of concussion and even of sudden death following a blow.

Here it is not necessary to do more than mention the fact that whereas the primary damage done to the brain, i.e. that inflicted at the moment of injury, is rarely fatal, death resulting from injury of the head is usually caused by secondary lesions such as swelling and displacement, with consequent hypoxia and infarction of the brain – the so-called second accident.

Open injuries

An open depressed fracture caused by localized impact and many penetrating injuries may do considerable damage to the brain but not cause the acceleration and deceleration that result in loss of consciousness. Although the damage done to the brain can be severe and quite extensive it is usually not diffuse, as it is with most closed injuries. This means that when the effects of local damage are clinically manifest they are physical rather than psychosocial in nature.

Penetration of the brain by missiles moving with high velocity is severely disruptive, with little or no prospect of survival. In this connection, it is interesting to note that if a high-velocity bullet passes through an empty skull it does little damage except where it enters and leaves the skull, but when there is a brain in the skull the former transmits the shock wave much more effectively than air does and the skull sustains extensive damage (R. Scott, personal communication).

Kidney

Closed injuries

The kidney may be damaged by impact from behind, in which case there may be associated fracture of a rib and injury of the spleen or the liver, or (by perhaps a slower and heavier blow) from in front. Although the renal capsule is usually torn by quite mild splits, the perinephric fascia often remains intact, with the result that, although there has been demonstrable escape of

blood and urine, the kidney often heals without lasting effect on its function. This means that if a surgeon finds a perinephric haematoma without obvious damage to the main blood vessels or the pelvis of the ureter, he will usually be well advised to leave it alone, unless there has been profuse and persistent haematuria. Exploring a perinephric haematoma can add accuracy to the diagnosis but at the possible cost of provoking troublesome bleeding, the control of which may result in further damage to the kidney.

Blood within the perinephric fascia needs to be distinguished from retroperitoneal blood that overlies the kidney but may have its source in a tear of the colon or the duodenum; such a possibility demands that the haematoma be explored.

Open injuries

Whether they are tidy or untidy, these resemble closed injuries in that, unless the damage is severe and extensive or affects the main blood vessels or the ureter, the kidney may heal without surgical intervention; however, it must be remembered that the main danger of such injuries arises from the fact that they may injure other important structures.

Suprarenal gland

All that needs to be said about this is that injuries are rare and, whether they are open or closed, their importance lies in the fact that they are likely to be associated with serious injuries of other viscera.

Liver and spleen

Closed injuries

As with the kidney, moderate force causes simple splits that can heal readily and without complication; modern radiological techniques have shown, contrary to previous beliefs, how well the spleen can heal. Heavier blows and crushing can shatter the organs, even to the extent of causing complete transection, which is likely to be because of being crushed against the spine. Bleeding is severe and persistent. In the case of the liver both deformation and displacement can tear the hepatic veins and even the inferior vena cava.

Both organs can suffer internal rupture. In the case of the spleen, subcapsular haematomata that burst through the capsule have been offered as the reason for delayed rupture of the organ, but it is open to question whether in the past it was the rupture or the diagnosis that was delayed.

In the liver, rupture sometimes occurs well inside the organ rather than near the capsule and, by tearing blood vessels and biliary ductules into a closed space, it sometimes causes haemobilia, which is characterized by upper abdominal pain, jaundice and melaena.

Open injuries

The importance of these depends upon the degree and extent of damage to the organs and their blood supply, the biliary tract and neighbouring organs.

Pancreas

Closed injuries

These result from blows in the epigastrium that catch the abdominal muscles off guard and are of sufficient force to crush the organ against the spine. The head may be crushed or the body transected but other organs may be displaced and so escape injury.

Open injuries

These are rare and serious; they are often accompanied by injuries of other organs. If they are not recognized early they can result in false cysts and fistulae.

Uterus

Except during pregnancy, the uterus is so small and tough that it is almost invulnerable, except by dilators, which can penetrate the wall with disconcerting ease.

During pregnancy the uterus can be regarded as a hollow organ but in spite of its large size for much of the time it is rarely injured by blows or penetrating injuries. Rupture of the pregnant uterus is usually the result of severe impact or crushing, which puts both the mother and the child in mortal peril. Occasionally a spike of bone in a broken pelvis will pierce the uterus, but not necessarily injure the fetus, whereas missiles are more likely to cause serious damage to the fetus than to the mother, whose abdominal viscera are kept out of the way.

Hollow organs

Lungs

Although most injuries of the lungs are open inasmuch as they affect the alveoli, the healthy lung rarely becomes infected after being injured.

Closed injuries

Impact may cause no more than subpleural bruising or superficial laceration by broken ribs, but heavier bows on a flexible chest wall, such as that of a child, can cause sufficient deformity to crush the hilum against the spine and transect it. Such an injury is not necessarily immediately fatal.

Blast. Although it may be tempting to regard blast as a form of impact it is, in fact, a disruptive process resulting from the passage of a shock wave generated by an explosion and there is nothing to add here to the description in Chapter 8.

Penetrating injuries

The lung is remarkably tolerant of penetrating injuries, which are serious when they affect large blood vessels, the tracheobronchial tree or vital organs. Even high-velocity missiles do relatively little damage to the lung itself. Apart from profuse bleeding, one of the most dramatic, and easily treatable, effects of injury of a lung is a valvular opening that leads to a rapidly expanding pneumothorax; it is not necessarily associated with surgical emphysema.

Larynx, trachea and bronchi

Injuries of the air passages are necessarily open injuries, as in the case of the lung, but 'closed' is here used to mean that the skin has not been broken.

Closed injuries

The larynx is fractured or it may be disconnected from the trachea by being driven against the spine. The combination of marks of impact with surgical emphysema in the neck strongly suggests that this has occurred, most probably in the course of a road accident.

The trachea can also be injured by impact in the neck. In old persons the hardened cartilages may be broken; in young persons the soft tissues between them can be torn, sometimes completely. In either case there may be obstructive swelling by bleeding as well as by surgical emphysema in the neck.

Although, as has been mentioned, the main bronchus can be severed by being crushed against the spine, severe deformation of the chest can stretch the bronchus sufficiently for it to tear more or less completely but without rupture of the blood vessels in the hilum of the lung. Depending on where the tear is, air will escape into the neck by way of the mediastinum or into the pleural cavity, and sometimes in both directions. Partial tears may be valvular.

Penetrating injuries

These are rare, whether they are caused from without by stabbing, shooting, accidental penetration or cutting the throat or, more probably, from within in the course of intubation.

Pharynx and oesophagus

The most likely cause of injury is by penetration, either from without or from within, by instruments or sharp swallowed objects. It is worth remembering that forcible penetration from without may extend as far as the spine, in which case there may be radiological evidence of damage to a vertebral body.

Rarely, fractures of the spine can damage these structures. Another rare cause of injury is massive and forcible vomiting or belching, which can split the oesophagus longitudinally near the cardia. Surgical emphysema or pneumothorax is likely to occur.

Stomach and bowel

Stomach

Rupture of the stomach is rare and usually longitudinal. Although it could conceivably result from being crushed against the spine, it is more likely to be caused by impact when the organ is distended, whether by gas or by food. The tear is usually anterior but both surfaces can be affected.

Penetration may be from without or by instruments or by sharp swallowed objects.

Duodenum

Rupture occurs as a result of crushing against the spine, where its relative fixity does not allow it to escape. The tear is usually transverse, but it may be anterior and intraperitoneal or posterior and extraperitoneal, in which case blood may be mixed with bile in surgical emphysema.

Less severe blows can cause an haematoma within the wall of the duodenum and it may be large enough to obstruct the lumen. Although it can be evacuated surgically, the swelling subsides within a few days and it may be possible to pass a feeding tube beyond, as well as keeping the stomach empty.

Small intestine

Closed injuries. In spite of its mobility, this can be crushed against the spine. The injuries range from subperitoneal haematoma, splitting of the peritoneal and muscular coats with herniation of the mucous membrane, to tearing of the full thickness of the wall and even transection. The bowel is sometimes torn from its mesentery and it may lose its blood supply as a result. Haematoma of the mesentery is often harmless but it can have a similar effect.

The bowel can be burst by a blast wave, as when there is an explosion under water with the victim in it. It can also be burst by a blow in the belly of a person with a hernia because the sudden rise in pressure tears the bowel where it lacks the support of the abdominal wall.

Penetrating injuries of the small bowel are rare and may occur from within or from without. Small holes such as are caused by shot-gun pellets may appear on casual inspection to be no more than sub-peritoneal petechiae, but there is usually a small surrounding area of oedema. They do not usually leak but should be repaired. Larger holes allow the mucous membrane to pout and there is more or less leakage of the contents.

Large intestine

Crushing. Only the transverse colon with its mesentery and the greater omentum are in danger of being crushed against the spine, but occasionally bowel is crushed against the inside of the iliac crest and I have known most of the right side of the colon to be reduced to a tube of mucosa, the main muscular layer having been split and then retracted completely. Impact against the lateral part of the posterior abdominal wall is likely to be less damaging because of the padding by muscles. It occasionally tears the colon, which is usually marked by a retroperitoneal haematoma. As mentioned in Chapter 8, bowel has been trapped in fractures of the pelvis.

Penetrating injuries. Stabbing and shooting may penetrate the trunk from any direction and may enter the abdominal cavity from quite a long way away. Accidental impalement can follow similar courses, including per anum; instruments and even enema tubes can do the same. A rare form of penetrating injury can follow a practical joke such as directing a jet of air under high pressure at the buttocks. The air can pass through clothing, enter the anus and burst the bowel.

Rectum

This part of the bowel can be injured in any of the above ways but it is subject to two peculiar injuries: one is being torn from its moorings and retracting into the pelvis when this is severely crushed, with consequent tearing asunder of the soft-tissue planes; the other is rupture by bursting in the course of a strenuous effort such as lifting. This is likely to occur if there is much gas in the rectum, which tears into the rectouterine or rectovesical pouch, where it is relatively unsupported.

Bladder

A full bladder can be burst by impact but whether it is full or empty it may be pierced by fragments of a broken pelvis. The former injuries are likely to be intraperitoneal and the latter extraperitoneal. Once the bladder is empty, the edges of the rent come together. It may well heal if the bladder is kept empty but repair adds welcome assurance about healing as well as about the state of the other viscera. A rare cause of penetration is pushing a guide wire too far when nailing a hip; such a puncture might be expected to heal if the bladder were kept empty but urine has been known to leak to the surface and one would need to be sure that the bowel had not been injured. In my experience of one such case, laparotomy while the wire was in place showed that it had pierced the peritoneum but had not harmed either the bowel or the bladder.

Vagina

Perhaps the commonest injury is tearing during delivery; in its most severe form it enters the anal canal. Violent sexual assault is another serious cause and in less reprehensible sexual activity, blowing into the vagina has been known to cause air embolism, but not necessarily with rupture of the structure. Severe fractures of the pelvis can involve the vagina in the disruption of the structures within the pelvis.

Other tubular structures

Biliary tract

The gall bladder can be torn, even completely avulsed. The former may be the result of direct impact; the latter, of violent displacement of the liver with consequent tearing of the peritoneum and the cystic duct. The degree of filling of the gall bladder may play a part in either of these injuries.

The bile ducts could conceivably be crushed against the spine or torn by stretching if the liver is violently displaced. They may also be injured by penetrating wounds, but the commonest cause of injury is a surgical accident.

Cisterna chyli and the lymphatic duct

Injuries are very rare, and less rare from penetrating wounds than from spikes of bone from the spine. Unless there has already been obvious effusion of chyle the lesion is easily overlooked in the course of exploration. Even when it is sought, it requires more than usual care, and perhaps luck, to identify the tear in such a small and collapsed structure surrounded by haematoma.

Ureter

Closed injuries of this tough and fairly easily displaceable tube are very rare and, except in the pelvis of the ureter, they are more likely to result from the stretching that accompanies violent distortion than from crushing. As with the biliary tract, the most frequent cause of injury is a surgical accident.

Urethra
Closed injuries

Rupture at the apex of the prostate usually occurs when the pubes are displaced backwards, but it is a moot point whether the urethra is torn by bone or by stretching. Although one might expect such injuries inevitably to be complete, my own experience matches that of the Bristol school in that, if immediate repair is not undertaken, it may be possible some days later to find a way into the bladder and to insert a catheter with the aid of a panendoscope. In the mean time, suprapubic drainage is used to keep the bladder empty. This suggests that rupture was incomplete.

Rupture by impact is even rarer and affects the bulbar part, which is crushed against the pubic arch. It is well known that such ruptures are often incomplete, but it is not well known that the narrow dorsal strip that maintains continuity of the urethra may be the entire circumference. In other words, in such a case the rupture has not been transverse but longitudinal and I have found it possible to draw the edges of the strip together and sew them up over a catheter.

Penetrating injuries

These are most likely to result from misdirected sounds or bougies, but the urethra is sometimes severed anywhere in its length by missiles.

Blood vessels
Aorta

Closed injuries, particularly during systole, could split the vessel longitudinally, but a more frequent cause of injury in the case of the thoracic aorta is traction such as occurs in the course of road accidents. This has been dealt with adequately in Chapter 8. Crush injuries of the abdominal aorta are usually below the renal arteries and the result of road accidents; they are not necessarily fatal (Lassonde and Laurendeau, 1981).

Open injuries. Injury by stabbing and gunshot and other missiles is often combined with injury of nearby organs but, if the victim reaches hospital alive, recovery may be possible. Some injuries of the aorta have bled into an adjoining organ such as the duodenum or the inferior vena cava (Dingledein *et al.*, 1977; Machiedo *et al.*, 1983). There have also been cases in which small bullets have caused self-sealing wounds and have become arterial emboli (Symbas and Harlaftis, 1977; Rich *et al.*, 1978). This condition should be suspected when there is no wound of exit and no sign of the bullet in the course it is likely to have taken (Yajko and Trimble, 1974). Pain may occur over a peripheral artery (Garzon and Gliedman, 1964).

Main pulmonary vessels

Closed injuries. Although, as has been mentioned on page 118, the main pulmonary vessels can be transected by crushing, less severe injuries can leave them in continuity even though the bronchus has been torn right through. In such a case, timely repair of the bronchus can restore normal function to the lung.

Penetrating injuries are particularly dangerous because of the proximity of other vital structures. Even though a missile stops short of these or other large blood vessels, if it is more than about half an inch (≈ 13 mm) across and is close to them, it should be removed lest infection, for example, should cause possibly fatal complications.

Great veins

Closed injuries, whether in the chest or the abdomen, are likely to be associated with injuries of such severity as to make survival unlikely.

Open injuries are rare. These days, penetrating injuries by misdirected catheters are perhaps the most frequent; they can result in intra- or extrapleural collections of one sort or another. Kirschner's wires have been known to break and become loose and work their way into large veins, and small bullets can cause self-sealing wounds and then move about under the influence of posture rather than the flow of blood. Sivanesan (1976) reported a case in which a bullet passed from an external iliac vein to the heart.

A particularly regrettable sort of injury has occurred during the surgical removal of an intervertebral disc (Holscher, 1968; Stokes, 1968). The accounts suggest that it can be disconcertingly easy to pierce the annulus fibrosus and damage an adjoining blood vessel. The right common iliac vein is particularly at risk.

Peripheral blood vessels

Closed injuries are usually associated with fractures where the vessels are close to bone. They may be caused by the force that breaks the bone or by fragments of the bone. The lesion ranges from mild bruising of the wall of the vessel to complete division, which latter may cause little bleeding because of the laceration and retraction of the vessel. In the case of an artery, an important intermediate stage is tearing of the intima, with perhaps no more than mild damage to the other two coats. The artery appears to be bruised at the site of injury, whereas it may in fact be occluded by a flap of intima, as a result of local swelling of the wall or by more or less spasm, in any combination. If there is only a poor collateral circulation the artery beyond the lesion is small and is liable to be thought to be in spasm, whereas, as a naturally contractile tube, it is simply not being filled to its usual size by blood. The vessel should be opened so that the appropriate repair can be carried out. If there is a good collateral circulation the distal part of the artery is likely to be filled with blood and to show pulsation. In such cases, repair has little advantage over ligation.

A rare injury is traumatic thrombosis of the ulnar artery in the palm, where a heavy blow or crushing can trap it against bone. The blood supply of the hand as a whole is usually well maintained by the palmar arches and their numerous anastomoses and the condition may be mistaken for damage to the nerve because of complaints of numbness and tingling.

In spite of the damage that can be caused in these ways, it is sometimes remarkable how the mobility of blood vessels within their sheaths of loose connective tissue can allow them to be displaced from danger.

Spasm. It is now well known that, although arteries do go into spasm, this is usually the result of stretching or the injection of an irritant substance, and is rarely the result of other damage.

Open injuries. In spite of the mobility of vascular and neurovascular bundles in their sheaths of loose connective tissue, they are quite often damaged by sharp and by blunt penetrating injuries. In most cases there is obvious need to explore the wound, but penetration by small objects such as shotgun pellets or slivers of glass or wire may seem to have done no serious damage until pain and swelling provide evidence of an arteriovenous fistula. This complication may also follow attempts at puncturing vessels.

Spinal cord and nerves

Spinal cord

Closed injuries

These are mostly the result of fractures and dislocations above the second lumbar vertebra. They may be inflicted either by translation at the fracture or by encroachment into the vertebral canal by bursting fractures. A similar effect can accompany backward herniation of an intervertebral disc. Another important cause of injury is compression between degenerate and bulging discs in front and infolded soft tissues behind, when an elderly or old neck is sharply extended, which has been described in Chapter 2.

The blood supply of the spinal cord comes largely from the anterior spinal artery and if this is injured the effect on the cord will extend beyond the site of injury. Another reason for increasing severity and extent of damage within the cord is extension of swelling and consequent ischaemia. One result of this is that paralysis that arises from the lower part of the cervical region and leaves the diaphragm (supplied by C3, 4 and 5) fully active can spread upwards by two or three segments and paralyse it, so making artificial ventilation necessary. Paralysis that has extended in this way cannot be relied upon to improve when the swelling subsides and, in spite of its popularity in some centres, there is no clear evidence that even very early decompression of the cord will either protect it or promote its recovery. If the cord is explored, one striking finding may be that it both looks and feels normal, even when there is complete paralysis.

Open injuries

Missile wounds of the spinal cord are unlikely to be followed by recovery but a near miss can lead to temporary paralysis – so-called concussion of the cord. Stab wounds of the cord are rare but have been used by those with the necessary anatomical knowledge and skill as a means of rendering a victim of robbery incapable of pursuit.

Although some regeneration of neurones within the spinal cord does occur, it is of no practical value.

Nerves

Closed injuries

Compression is a frequent cause of the temporary paralyses such as having one's arm 'go to sleep', foot drop after sitting with the legs crossed in a way that squeezes the common peroneal nerve against the neck of the fibula and the so-called Saturday night paralysis of the radial nerve caused by prolonged pressure during drunken stupor. These are examples of neurapraxia, in which there is little or no structural damage to the nerve – anoxia may be solely responsible and recovery is complete, even within a matter of minutes.

The next order of damage is axonotmesis, in which the axon is interrupted within an unbroken myelin sheath. This can be likened to squashing an uncooked sausage between the fingers. When the axon regenerates it grows down its own sheath and, unless this takes so long that the end-organs degenerate, recovery will be complete.

The third order of damage is neurotmesis, in which sheaths as well as axons are interrupted and this may vary from partial to complete division of the nerve. Severe local crushing sometimes divides the whole nerve except for its epineurium and may be mistaken for a lesion in continuity with bruising. Recovery from neurotmesis is necessarily slow and often incomplete, even after the most careful surgical repair.

Many of the more serious closed lesions have a mixture of these three grades of injury with the result that, after some early recovery, there is a variable interval before any more takes place.

Acute compression follows a blow where a nerve is fairly near the surface and also close to bone. Tourniquet paralysis is a cause of acute compression in which the damage is anoxic neurapraxia.

Chronic compression is most familiar as the carpal tunnel syndrome; the tarsal tunnel syndrome is much less frequent. Many conditions have been described in which fibrous bands press on nerves such as the anterior and the posterior interosseous nerves in the upper part of the forearm. Cysts and tumours near or within nerves may also be responsible. In such cases there may be sufficient scarring within to prevent full recovery when the cause of pressure has been removed.

Traction. Any force that greatly increases the distance between the origin of a nerve and its termination will stretch it beyond its elastic limit and cause a combination of axonotmesis and neurotmesis. If it is sufficiently severe, traction will tear nerves, perhaps in continuity, and even avulse them from the spinal cord, in which case subsequent myelography shows saccular extensions of the subarachnoid space. Whether or not avulsion does occur, the damage affects a considerable length of the nerve(s) concerned.

Traction and compression. If traction occurs while a nerve is passing over or round a bony prominence, the damage may be concentrated there and combine traction with compression. Examples include damage to the lower trunk of the brachial plexus, as in Klumpke's paralysis in the newborn and if a steep Trendelenburg position is used in a paralysed patient. Even more familiar is damage to the axillary nerve in the course of dislocation of the shoulder. Traction and compression combined with friction are responsible for the late ulnar palsy in cases of marked cubitus valgus.

Traction and compression over sharp edges of broken bone can inflict serious damage on nerves such as the radial, the sciatic at the hip joint and the common peroneal at the neck of the fibula. Damage of this sort is fortunately rare and most closed injuries accompanying fractures recover spontaneously.

Open injuries

Any nerves can be damaged by penetrating injuries, whether by sharp or blunt objects but, like blood vessels, their displaceability can protect them remarkably well.

References

Brash, J. C. (1955) *Neurovascular Hila of Limb Muscles*. E. and S. Livingstone, Edinburgh and London

Dingledein, G. P., Proctor, H. J. and Jaques, P. F. (1977) Traumatic aorto-caval-portal-duodenal fistula. *Journal of Trauma*, **17**, 474

Garzon, A. and Gliedman, M. L. (1964) Peripheral embolization of a bullet following perforation of the thoracic aorta. *Annals of Surgery*, **160**, 190

Gurdjian, E. S. (1971) Mechanisms of impact injury of the head. In *Proceedings of an International Symposium, Edinburgh and Madrid; April, 1970,* Churchill Livingstone, Edinburgh and London

Holbourn, A. H. S. (1945) Mechanics of head injuries. *British Medical Bulletin*, **3**, 147

Holscher, E. C. (1968) Vascular and visceral injuries during lumbar-disc surgery. *Journal of Bone and Joint Surgery*, **50A**, 383

Lassonde, J. and Laurendeau, F. (1981) Blunt injury of the abdominal aorta. *Annals of Surgery*, **194**, 745

Machiedo, G. W., Jain, K. M., Swan, K. G., Petrocelli, J. C. and Blackwood, J. M. (1983) Traumatic aorto-caval fistula. *Journal of Trauma*, **23**, 243

Pudenz, R. H. and Sheldon, C. H. (1946) The lucite calvarium – a method for direct observation of the brain. *Journal of Neurosurgery*, **3**, 487

Rich, N. M., Collins, G. J., Anderson, C. A., McDonald, P. T., Kozloff, L. and Ricotta, J. J. (1978) Missile emboli. *Journal of Trauma*, **18**, 236

Sivanesan, S. (1976) Bullet embolism to the heart. *Medicine, Science and the Law*, **16**, 59

Stokes, J. M. (1968) Vascular complications of disc surgery. *Journal of Bone and Joint Surgery*, **50A**, 394

Strich, S. J. (1961) Shearing of nerve fibres as a cause of brain damage due to head injury. Lancet, **ii**, 443

Symbas, P. M. and Harlaftis, N. (1977) Bullet emboli in the pulmonary and systemic arteries. *Annals of Surgery*, **185**, 318

Yajko, D. and Trimble, C. (1974) Arterial bullet embolism following abdominal gunshot wounds. *Journal of Trauma*, **14**, 200

Index